Judith Buddensiek

Influence of Cerebrospinal fluid on the behaviour of neural stem cells

Judith Buddensiek

Influence of Cerebrospinal fluid on the behaviour of neural stem cells

An in vitro study

Südwestdeutscher Verlag für Hochschulschriften

Impressum/Imprint (nur für Deutschland/only for Germany)
Bibliografische Information der Deutschen Nationalbibliothek: Die Deutsche Nationalbibliothek verzeichnet diese Publikation in der Deutschen Nationalbibliografie; detaillierte bibliografische Daten sind im Internet über http://dnb.d-nb.de abrufbar.
Alle in diesem Buch genannten Marken und Produktnamen unterliegen warenzeichen-, marken- oder patentrechtlichem Schutz bzw. sind Warenzeichen oder eingetragene Warenzeichen der jeweiligen Inhaber. Die Wiedergabe von Marken, Produktnamen, Gebrauchsnamen, Handelsnamen, Warenbezeichnungen u.s.w. in diesem Werk berechtigt auch ohne besondere Kennzeichnung nicht zu der Annahme, dass solche Namen im Sinne der Warenzeichen- und Markenschutzgesetzgebung als frei zu betrachten wären und daher von jedermann benutzt werden dürften.

Coverbild: www.ingimage.com

Verlag: Südwestdeutscher Verlag für Hochschulschriften GmbH & Co. KG
Heinrich-Böcking-Str. 6-8, 66121 Saarbrücken, Deutschland
Telefon +49 681 37 20 271-1, Telefax +49 681 37 20 271-0
Email: info@svh-verlag.de

Approved by: Greifswald, EMAU, Diss., 2011

Herstellung in Deutschland:
Schaltungsdienst Lange o.H.G., Berlin
Books on Demand GmbH, Norderstedt
Reha GmbH, Saarbrücken
Amazon Distribution GmbH, Leipzig
ISBN: 978-3-8381-3082-8

Imprint (only for USA, GB)
Bibliographic information published by the Deutsche Nationalbibliothek: The Deutsche Nationalbibliothek lists this publication in the Deutsche Nationalbibliografie; detailed bibliographic data are available in the Internet at http://dnb.d-nb.de.
Any brand names and product names mentioned in this book are subject to trademark, brand or patent protection and are trademarks or registered trademarks of their respective holders. The use of brand names, product names, common names, trade names, product descriptions etc. even without a particular marking in this works is in no way to be construed to mean that such names may be regarded as unrestricted in respect of trademark and brand protection legislation and could thus be used by anyone.

Cover image: www.ingimage.com

Publisher: Südwestdeutscher Verlag für Hochschulschriften GmbH & Co. KG
Heinrich-Böcking-Str. 6-8, 66121 Saarbrücken, Germany
Phone +49 681 37 20 271-1, Fax +49 681 37 20 271-0
Email: info@svh-verlag.de

Printed in the U.S.A.
Printed in the U.K. by (see last page)
ISBN: 978-3-8381-3082-8

Copyright © 2012 by the author and Südwestdeutscher Verlag für Hochschulschriften GmbH & Co. KG and licensors
All rights reserved. Saarbrücken 2012

Table of contents

1. Introduction — 3
1.1 Neurodegenerative disorders — 3
1.2 Cell therapy in Parkinson´s disease — 4
1.3 Neural Stem cells: Origins — 6
1.4 Neural stem cells: Definition — 7
1.5 Cerebrospinal Fluid — 8
1.6 Aim of the studies — 10

2. Material and Methods — 11

3. Results — 12

4. Discussion — 14

5. Summary — 17

6. References — 19

7. Appendices — 22
7.1 Acknowledgements — 22
7.2 Referred publications — 23

1. Introduction

1.1 Neurodegenerative disorders

The term neurodegenerative disorders denotes all chronic disorders leading to a progressive loss of structure or function of neurons or glial cells in the brain or spinal cord. These neurodegenerative processes can either be localized or diffuse, and they may affect a single or even multiple neuronal systems such as the motor or sensory system, or the cerebral cortex. Neurodegenerative disorders are classified according to their topographic distribution and their aetiology.

Examples of important diseases belonging to the neurodegenerative disorders are Huntington's disease (HD), Amyotrophic lateral sclerosis (ALS), Alzheimer's disease (DAT) and Parkinson's disease (PD) [1, 2]. To date, all neurodegenerative disorders remain incurable and all available treatments aim to improve the functional capacity of the patient and to slow down the progression of the neurodegenerative process without being able to inhibit it. However, over the past two decades, cell replacement therapies have been proposed as a potentially new approach to restore the damaged and dysfunctional brain regions, aiming to induce a long-lasting clinical improvement or even recovery [2].

1.2 Cell therapy in Parkinson's disease

One of the most common neurodegenerative disorders is PD, affecting an increasing number of more than four million people worldwide [3]. PD is caused by a selective degeneration of dopaminergic neurons in the substantia nigra (SNR), a part of the midbrain (Fig.1).

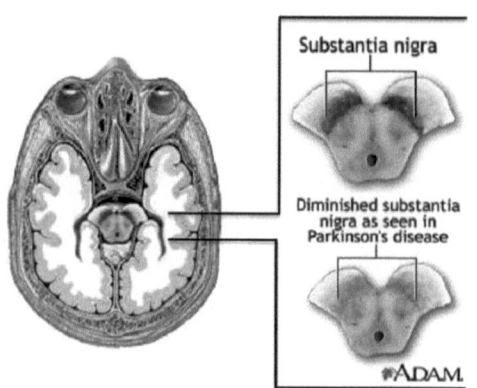

Fig. 1:

Degenerative loss of dopaminergic cells in the substantia nigra, part of the midbrain, in Parkinson's Disease.

(Picture modified from:
http://mirrorreflections.files.wordpress.com/2008/09/parkinsons-disease-affected-brain-deaconess-do-tcom.jpg, march 2010)

Early on motor symptoms such as bradykinesia, rigidity, resting tremor and unstable posture tend to predominate. As the condition progresses non-motor symptoms such as vegetative disorders, deterioration of cognition or psychiatric disturbances [4, 5] emerge. To date, PD is symptomatically treated with dopamine precursors or agonists, aiming to substitute the loss of dopamine in the STN. However, these agents have a large side effect profile and patients often become tolerant to them, frequently suffering from episodes of "freezing", fluctuations in motor response, involuntary movements or dyskinesias after long-term administration [2, 6]. Contrary to this, the administration of long-acting dopamine agonists such as bromocriptine or ropinerole lead to a lower incidence of dyskinesia [7] but increases the risk of psychotic symptoms in elderly PD patients with dementia [8]. Additionally, the occurrence of adverse events such as leg oedema, daytime somnolence, impulse control disorders and fibrosis has recently been highlighted during administration of dopamine agonists in PD patients [9]. Because of the rather selective degeneration of the nigrostriatal dopamine system, PD seems to be particularly amenable to cell replacement therapies, which is why the transplantation of human fetal ventral mesencephalic tissues into the striatum of late-stage PD patients has been adopted in clinical trials since the late 1980s [10, 11]. To date, more than 350 patients with PD have successfully received intrastriatal implants leading to a clinical benefit, which for some has even resulted in the withdrawal of L-Dopa medication for several years. The robust survival, integration and functioning of the implants can be proven by postoperative PET-Scans, which show a massively increased ^{18}Fluorodopa tracer uptake, and also by post-mortem analyses of transplanted patients [11-14]. However, the fetal tissue transplantation shows a large variability of functional outcomes, with troublesome dyskinesias occurring in a significant proportion of the grafted patients, which is thought to be the result of an excessive, heterogenous dopaminergic innervation provided by the implant. Furthermore, there are ethical and logistic problems of acquiring fetal tissues and beside the standard surgical risks, the intrastriatal implantation causes extended tissue damage at the implantation site(s). For these reasons several scientific issues still need to be addressed before cell replacement therapies may become a real therapeutic option in neurodegenerative disorders such as PD [11-13].

1.3 Neural Stem cells: Origins

Neural stem cells (NSCs) have been defined as multipotent derivates of the neuroectodermal tissue, having the capacity to self-renew and to give rise to all cells of the three major neural phenotypes (astrocytes, oligodendrocytes and neurons) via lineage-restricted precursor cells. In contrast to the pluripotent embryonic stem (ES) cells they are thus more restricted in their differentiation capacity and therefore lack the risk of tumor formation after transplantation. This is one of the reasons why NSCs present a promising source for cell replacement therapies of the central nervous system (CNS).

NSCs can either be directly extracted from fetal nervous tissue or isolated from different regions of the adult brain, such as the subventricular zone (SVZ), the hippocampus, the lateral ventricles and some nonneurogenic regions such as the spinal cord [15].

Additionally, NSCs can be generated from ES cells, which are pluripotent cells, isolated from the inner cell mass of the preimplantation blastocyst that can give rise to cell lineages of any type of body tissue from all three embryonic germ layers. However, they are not totipotent, because they fail to develop a whole functional organism. Unfortunately, there is a high risk of tumor formation after the transplantation of ES cells [16] because of their uncontrollable proliferation potential in vivo [17, 18] and the occurrence of chromosomal aberrations, common in long-term maintained ES cells in culture [19].

Furthermore, it has recently been reported, that NSCs can also be generated from multipotent adult stem cells of other tissues, which are able to break barriers of germ layer commitment to transdifferentiate into neuroectodermal cell types. This finding is of great importance for autologous transplantation approaches [20-23] (Fig. 2).

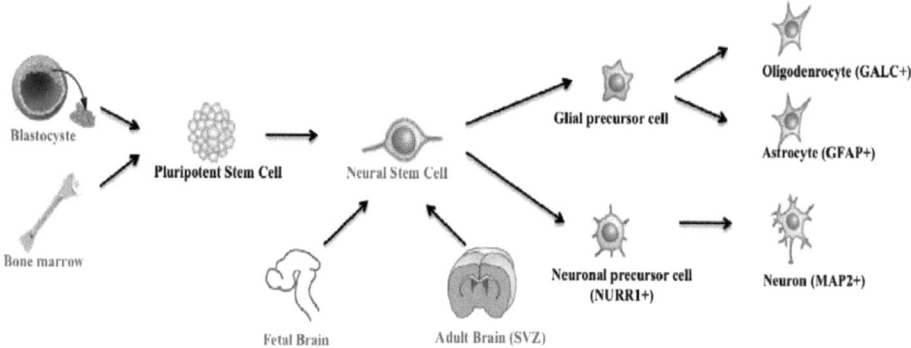

Fig. 2: Schematic overview of various sources of NSCs, with the capacity to differentiate into the three major neural phenotypes namely oligodendrocytes, astrocytes and neurons.

The NSCs used in our studies were directly extracted from rat embryonic mesencephalic tissue or isolated from the hippocampal region of the human adult brain.

1.4 Neural stem cells: Definition

As mentioned above, NSCs are defined as multipotent cells derived from the neuroectodermal tissue, having the capacity to regenerate and to differentiate into all cells of the three major neural phenotypes: astrocytes, oligodendrocytes and neurons. Beyond theory, NSCs are often identified by their behaviour after isolation. During expansion, they usually grow in floating, multicellular aggregates, so-called "neurospheres". Attempts have been made to develop markers to define NSCs but they have often been discarded again because they were found to also be expressed on non-neuronal cells [15]. Nevertheless, commercially available fetal neural progenitor cells could recently be characterized by Vogel et al. as CD15, CD56, CD90, CD133, CD164, CD172a, nerve growth factor receptor NGFR, W4A5 and 57D2 positive, while negative for CD45, CD105 (endoglin), CD109, CD140b (PDGF-RB) and W8B2 [24]. In addition, an extensive analysis of surface markers on clonogenic human fetal neurosphere cultures was performed by Uchida et al., defining a subset of human NSCs as phenotypically CD133-positive, but negative for CD34 and CD45 [25]. Furthermore, the expression of specific neural transcription factors, such as Sox-1, Musashi-1, Otx-1, Otx-2, Neurod1 and neurogenin-2 was reported in fetal neural stem and progenitor cells, demonstrating their neuroectodermal origin [26]. Still, most of the studies attempting to characterize NSCs have been performed with non-human mammalian hippocampal NSCs, whereas very little is known about their human counterparts. The most likely explanation for this is the lack of tissue availability.

1.5 Cerebrospinal Fluid

The adult CNS is surrounded by approximately 140 ml of cerebrospinal fluid (CSF), which is replaced every 5-9 hours. CSF is generated in the "choroid plexus" which is situated in the lateral, third and fourth ventricles of the brain. CSF circulation takes place from the brain cavities down to the brain stem and spinal cord or to the subarachnoid space and further toward the parasaggital region where re-absorption occurs (Fig.3).

Normal CSF is a crystal-clear fluid, mainly composed of water (99%), but also containing common solutes such as Sodium, Potassium, Glucose and Lactate, CNS-specific and serum derived proteins and a small number of cells, mostly lymphocytes and monocytes [27]. CSF composition varies between lumbar and ventricular CSF as a consequence of passive diffusion processes across the blood-CSF-barrier. Also active secretion processes during the cranio-caudal circulation have to be considered [28]. Additionally, CSF can be pathologically modified in neurodegenerative disorders such as PD and ALS with markedly increased levels of proinflammatory prostaglandins such as PGE_2 and cytokines such as TNF-α, interferon-β and IL-1b [15].

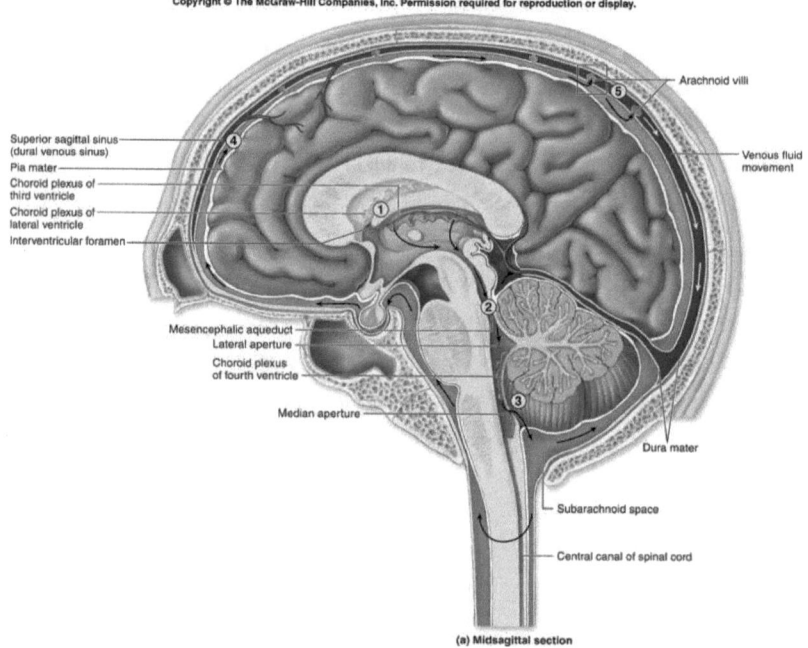

Fig. 3: Schematic overview of CSF circulation and resorption.

(Picture modified from: http://academic.kellogg.edu/her-brandsonc/bio201_McKinley/f15-8b_production_and_c_c.jpg, march 2010)

Physiological functions of CSF include the protection of the brain during blood pressure fluctuations, the regulation of the chemical environment of the central nervous system, defence against pathogen invasion, intracerebral transport of biomolecules and removal of CNS metabolites [27]. Furthermore, several studies recently postulated that diffusible factors in embryonic CSF as well as CSF circulation and pressure regulate survival, differentiation and proliferation of neuroectodermal stem cells and reported on the pivotal importance of CSF in brain development in vivo.

Concerning the CSF components responsible for CSF influence on the basic behavioural parameters of NSCs, most studies so far concentrated on proteins (such as transthyretin, serin, retinol binding protein, heparan sulfate, several apolipoproteins, bone morphogenic protein), "membranous particles", amino acids and growth factors such as FGF2. Still, most of these studies have been performed with embryonic CSF, which is known to be much more complex in its protein composition than adult CSF. Conclusions for adult CSF influence on neuroectodermal stem cells and brain development should therefore be cautiously made, although it is known that adult NSCs of the SVZ have transitory contact with the ventricular brain cavities, which may also suggest regulatory effects of adult CSF on adult NSCs [15, 28].

1.6 Aim of the studies

As already mentioned above, intracerebral surgical cell transplantation in neurodegenerative disorders always involves surgical risks and tissue damage at the transplantation site(s) in an already damaged and dysfunctional brain [12]. Therefore alternative stem cell transplantation via CSF has been investigated recently, for example in animal models of spinal cord injured rats or ALS mice. In the spinal cord injured rat models, intensive invasion, migration, and integration of the transplanted NSCs into the damaged spinal cord have been detected after cell transplantation via CSF. Contrary to this, there has been no sufficient migration of intrathecally applied neuroectodermally converted human bone marrow-derived mesodermal stromal cells (hMSC-NSCs) into the CNS in an ALS mouse model which aimed to delay the first signs of disease or to prolong the survival of the mice. As a possible explanation for this finding a low survival rate of the applied cells due to the low nutrition content of CSF was discussed. Interestingly, so far most studies investigating the influence of CSF contents on survival, proliferation and differentiation of neural cell types were performed with embryonic avian CSF even though there are well-known differences between avian and mammalian CSF [15].

The scope of my thesis was to investigate the effects of adult human CSF on adult human (ahNSCs) and fetal murine (fmNSCs) neural stem cells in an attempt to answer the following questions:

1.) Does human adult CSF decrease the survival rate of ahNSCs and fmNSCs compared to standard culture media?
2.) Does human adult CSF influence the stem cell potential of ahNSCs and fmNSCs compared to standard culture media?
3.) Does human adult CSF influence the cell extension outgrowth velocity in ahNSCs and fmNSCs compared to standard differentiation media?
4.) Does human adult CSF influence the differentiation and gene expression of ahNSCs and fmNSCs compared to standard differentiation media?

In doing so, the ultimate aim has been to determine whether adult human CSF influences NSCs in a way, making it a limiting factor for a non-traumatic cell transplantation via CSF in patients with neurodegenerative disorders.

2. Material and Methods

For our studies, we collected adult human leptomeningeal cerebrospinal fluid from Idiopathic Normal Pressure Hydrocephalus patients, using lumbar puncture [15, 28].
Adult human hippocampal tissue for isolation and propagation of ahNSCs was obtained from routine epilepsy surgical procedures [28].
Fetal murine mesencephalic tissue for isolation and propagation of fmNSCs was obtained from E14.5 rat embryonic brain, being prepared according to standard procedures [15].
AhNSCs and fmNSCs were cultured in standard culture media KO-DMEM/EM1, supplemented with growth factors EGF and FGF, or CSF respectively, at 37°C in a humidified atmosphere and lowered O_2 conditions. During the differentiation process cells were plated onto poly-L-lysine-coated chamber slides or 6-well-plates in P4-8F differentiation medium or CSF without addition of any growth factors. Some of the differentiation experiments were conducted in the presence of the Bone Morphogenic Protein (BMP) inhibitor Noggin.
For determining the survival rate during expansion and differentiation, the self-renewing capacity and cell fate decisions immuncytochemistry was carried out using standard protocols [15, 28]. Additionally RNA extraction and quantitative RT-PCR analysis were performed [15].

3. Results

In our studies we investigated the influence of adult human CSF on survival and differentiation behaviour of ahNSCs and fmNSCs.

We found, that CSF enhances significantly the survival of both, ahNSCs and fmNSCs after expansion for 24 hours and differentiation for 24 and 72 hours, compared to standard culture media KO-DMEM or EM1 [15, 28].

Concerning the proliferation potential of ahNSCs and fmNSCs, we observed an inhibiting effect of CSF, leading to an accelerated loss of self-renewing capacity compared to standard expansion media, 24 and 72 hours after starting expansion process [15, 28].

Additionally, we found an enhancing effect of CSF on the extension outgrowth velocity of NSCs. In fmNSCs, CSF lead to significantly longer and a significantly larger number of cell extensions compared to standard differentiation media P4-8F during the first hours after starting the differentiation process [15]. In ahNSCs, the final length of cell extensions was more than twice as long in CSF compared to standard differentiation media and a significantly larger number of cell extensions could be determined from 6 hours after starting the differentiation process [28].

Concerning the CSF influence on cell fate decision we determined an astrogliogenesis facilitating effect on ahNSCs and fmNSCs with significantly more GFAP+ cells in CSF compared to standard differentiation media after 7-14 days of differentiation [15, 28]. While we also found an inhibiting effect on neurogenesis in fmNSCs with significantly less MAP+ and GALC+ cells in CSF compared to standard differentiation media [15], we observed no significant influence on the percentage of neurones and oligodendrocytes in ahNSCs. Still, we found significantly more Tubulin III+, immature neurons, in standard differentiation media compared to CSF in ahNSCs [28].

CSF effects on gene expression during the first 72 hours of differentiation were investigated in fmNSCs. According to our findings in immuncytochemistry after differentiation for 7-14 days, we observed a continuous increase in GFAP mRNA during the whole observation period with a significant higher increase in GFAP mRNA at 6 hours after starting the differentiation process in CSF compared to standard differentiation media. Additionally, a significantly higher expression of Nestin mRNA could be determined in CSF compared to standard differentiation media at 3 and 6 hours after starting the differentiation process and only in standard differentiation media did we find a significant decrease of Nestin mRNA under the initial value at 72 hours after starting the differentiation process. Concerning the TUBB mRNA expression we could not observe any significant influence of CSF [15].

The reversibility of CSF effects on fmNSCs and ahNSCs was tested using the BMP inhibitor Noggin [15, 28]. In fmNSCs, addition of Noggin reversed completely the survival enhancing effects of CSF during expansion for 72 and differentiation for 24 hours. Also, the influence of CSF on the extension outgrowth velocity was partly reversed by Noggin, with significantly shorter cell extensions at 3 hours and a significantly smaller number of cell extensions at 3, 6 and 12 hours after starting the differentiation process. Additionally, CSF effects on self-renewing capacity observed with Ki67 staining were inhibited by Noggin [15].

In ahNSCs, addition of Noggin did not significantly influence cell death rates during expansion for 72 and differentiation for 24 hours compared to CSF without Noggin [28].

4. Discussion

The central finding of our studies is that, in vitro, adult human leptomeningeal CSF promotes survival, differentiation and astrogliogenesis in ahNSCs and fmNSCs. A low survival rate of intrathecally applied NSCs due to a low nutrition content of CSF, as discussed by Habisch et al., therefore seems improbable [15, 28]. Still, adult human leptomeningeal CSF leads to a quicker loss of stem cell potential and enhances extension outgrowth velocity. This may cause an attachment of injected NSCs at the wall of the ventricle were they are injected and impede sufficient migration into the CNS [15]. Additionally, CSF promotes astrogliogenesis and in fmNSCs even inhibits the differentiation into neurons [15, 28]. This may also be a disadvantageous CSF effect, impeding intracerebral NSC differentiation into the required neurons after non-traumatic NSCs transplantation. The CSF components responsible for these effects on NSCs have not yet been sufficiently investigated but we found BMPs to be at least partly involved in CSF effects on fmNSCs. Some of these BMP effects could in vitro be blocked by Noggin [15], but in vivo experiments investigating the influence of Noggin on intrathecally injected NSCs are missing. Future studies are needed to gain deeper knowledge about CSF contents, their influence on NSCs and ways of controlling them before intrathecally NSC transplantation may become a functional alternative for surgical transplantation methods. Additionally, changes in CSF composition have to be considered in patients with neurodegenerative disorders and it is not yet clear what effects pathologically modified human CSF may have on intrathecally injected NSCs. Studying the influence of pathological human CSF on NSCs might be an interesting objective for further investigations.

Irrespective of the mode of transplantation, doubts recently arose about tissue transplantation as a potentially curative approach in neurodegenerative disorders. There are several reasons for this. The first is that several recent studies reported the degeneration of implanted cells, similar to the degeneration of endogenous neurons in the same pathological area, questioning the long-term efficacy of stem cell transplantation. Li et al. and Kordower et al. performed post mortem analysis of PD patients 10 years after fetal tissue transplantation and found pathological changes associated with PD, i.e. Lewy bodies (LB), in implanted surviving dopaminergic neurons suggesting host-to-graft disease propagation [29-31]. Similar results have been found in HD patients 18 months after they underwent neural transplantation, with disease-like neuronal degeneration and a preferential loss of projection neurons being seen [32]. Still, the effect of pathological changes like LB on the function of grafted neurons is unclear since there are no clinical or PET follow-up studies of patients beyond one decade after transplantation. Furthermore, the mechanism underlying the propagation of PD pathology from diseased to healthy transplanted neurons remains uncertain and several hypothesis from inflammation over oxidative stress, loss of neurotrophic support and prion-disease-like mechanisms are discussed [33]. Nevertheless, there is mounting evidence for an ongoing pathology in neurodegenerative disorders, also affecting transplanted neurons long term. Whether a permanent cure in patients with neurodegenerative disorders may be achieved with cell replacement therapies is therefore doubtable. Instead, a combination of cell replacement therapies with strategies to hinder disease progression seems to be required.

Another reason for doubting the approach of cell replacement therapies in neurodegenerative disorders is the growing evidence of so far maybe underestimated and not sufficiently explored self-repair mechanisms of the adult mammalian brain. They may offer several advantages over other cell based treatment strategies: immunological reactions and surgical procedures are circumvented and the ethical issues surrounding the use of ES cells are avoided. As mentioned above, neurogenesis in the SVZ and the hippocampal region of the adult mammalian brain has long been recognised [15] and the effects of brain pathology such as ischemia or hypoxia and of distinct growth factors on adult neurogenesis have been investigated. As reviewed by Lindvall et al. adequate blood supply seems to be crucial for adult neurogenesis, and angiogenesis in the adult brain after stroke seems to be closely associated with this. Administration of vascular endothelial growth factor (VEGF) further enhanced this effect [34]. In other studies, application of distinct growth factors such as nerve growth factor (NGF), brain derived neurotrophic factor (BDNF), neurotrophin 4/5, glial cell line-derived neurotrophic factor (GDNF) and epidermal growth factor (EGF) has been reported to promote survival and differentiation of specific neural subpopulations in vitro and in vivo [35]. GDNF has additionally been proposed as an interesting candidate for combination with cell replacement therapies [36]. The fact that SVZ precursors seem to be amenable to external modulation, makes them a potential therapeutic target to replace neuronal densities and circuitry in neurodegenerative disorders such as PD [37]. Still, most recent studies on endogenous dopaminergic regeneration in PD models aimed at using SVZ NSCs, driving them to migrate into the striatum and to differentiate into dopaminergic neurons. This seems necessary since there is so far no evidence for orthopic striatal dopaminergic neurogenesis. However, dopaminergic neurons generated from SVZ precursors constitute a different population of dopaminergic neurons that only share few characteristics with midbrain dopaminergic neurons affected in PD and there is so far no clear correlation between dopaminergic differentiation and functional recovery in animal models of PD. This is why neurogenesis restoring the dopamine deficit within the striatum has not yet been conclusively demonstrated. Further understanding about the cell-intrinsic restrictions of precursors from different brain regions is needed to be able to overcome these local commitments and to restore the nigrostriatal dopaminergic system by endogenous neurogenesis [37, 38].

Finally, advances in surgical treatment of neurodegenerative disorders, especially in PD, have to be considered and markedly increase requirements for new therapeutic approaches such as cell replacement therapies. Deep brain stimulation (DBS), for example, is adjustable and reversible and the surgical treatment of choice in PD patients with motor complications that cannot be adequately managed with medication. Recently, the first randomized controlled trial of patients receiving either DBS or best medical treatment has been published, proving DBS to be more effective in improving motor function, including the troublesome dyskinesias and quality of life at six months. Still DBS was associated with an increased risk of serious adverse events due to the surgical procedure, stimulation device or stimulation therapy [39]. This is the reason why benefits and risk of DBS still have to be carefully weighted and why DBS, though being an effective surgical PD treatment, still remains reserved for selected PD patients.

Summing up it can be said that neurodegenerative disorders lead to a continuous loss of structure or function of nerve cells in the central nervous system [2] and while they continue to gain in importance in an ageing society there is still no restoring therapy available [2, 3]. Nevertheless several potential therapeutic approaches have been discussed in the recent years, including the transplantation of developing neural tissue or NSCs into the damaged CNS and the induction of proliferation and migration of endogenous NSCs [37, 38, 40]. Still, the question of the clinical usefulness of these approaches has so far not been conclusively answered and many challenges have to be overcome before any of them may be applied to patients. One of these challenges is to avoid invasive surgical procedures containing surgical risks and damages of already dysfunctional tissue in cell replacement therapies. This is why we investigated the influence of CSF on NSCs in vitro aiming to gain deeper knowledge about possible limitations of non-traumatic transplantation of NSCs via CSF. In the end, the clinical usefulness of all new therapeutic approaches and transplantation methods will be determined by their ability to counteract disease progression and to provide patients with neurological disorders with safe, long-lasting and significant clinical improvements in quality of life.

5. Summary

Neurodegenerative disorders are characterized by a progressive loss of structure or function of neurons or glial cells in the brain or spinal cord. Thus, the prospect of replacing the missing or damaged nerve tissue is very attractive. A promising source for cell replacement therapies for neurodegenerative disorders are neural stem cells (NSCs).

As an alternative to the intracerebral stereotactical surgical cell transplantation, the administration of NSCs via cerebrospinal fluid (CSF) has recently been proposed as a non- traumatic transplantation method into the brain. However, cell survival and intraparenchymal migration of the transplants were limited. As a possible reason the low nutrition content of CSF was discussed. Furthermore, CSF was recently reported to be an important milieu for controlling stem cell processes in the developing brain, which is why we studied the effects of adult human leptomeningeal CSF on the behaviour of fetal murine (fmNSCs) and adult human NSCs (ahNSCs).

The central findings of our studies are that, in vitro, adult human leptomeningeal CSF:

(i)   enhances the survival rate of ahNSCs and fmNSCs during expansion and differentiation compared to standard culture/differentiation media
(ii) enhances NSC differentiation and extension outgrowth velocity, leading to a faster loss of self-renewing capacity
(iii) has an astrogliogenesis facilitating effect on ahNSCs and fmNSCs and inhibits neurogenesis in fmNSCs.

A low survival rate of intrathecally applied NSCs due to a low nutrition content of CSF therefore seems improbable. Still, adult human leptomeningeal CSF leads to a quicker loss of stem cell potential and enhances extension outgrowth velocity. This may cause an attachment of injected NSCs at the wall of the ventricle where they are injected and impede sufficient migration into the CNS. Additionally, CSF promotes astrogliogenesis and in fmNSCs even inhibits the differentiation into neurons. This may also be a disadvantageous CSF effect, impeding intracerebral NSC differentiation into required neurons after non-traumatic NSCs transplantation.

For these reasons, future studies are demanded to gain deeper knowledge about CSF contents, their influence on NSCs and ways of controlling them before intrathecally NSC transplantation may become a functional alternative to surgical transplantation methods.

6. References

1. Martin JB: **Molecular basis of the neurodegenerative disorders.** *The New England journal of medicine* 1999, **340**(25):1970-1980.
2. Moon BS, Yoon JY, Kim MY, Lee SH, Choi T, Choi KY: **Bone morphogenetic protein 4 stimulates neuronal differentiation of neuronal stem cells through the ERK pathway.** *Experimental & molecular medicine* 2009, **41**(2):116-125.
3. Dorsey ER, Constantinescu R, Thompson JP, Biglan KM, Holloway RG, Kieburtz K, Marshall FJ, Ravina BM, Schifitto G, Siderowf A et al: **Projected number of people with Parkinson disease in the most populous nations, 2005 through 2030.** *Neurology* 2007, **68**(5):384-386.
4. Gupta A, Dawson TM: **The role of stem cells in Parkinson's disease.** *Neurosurgery clinics of North America* 2007, **18**(1):129-142, x-xi.
5. Hodaie M, Neimat JS, Lozano AM: **The dopaminergic nigrostriatal system and Parkinson's disease: molecular events in development, disease, and cell death, and new therapeutic strategies.** *Neurosurgery* 2007, **60**(1):17-28; discussion 28-30.
6. Ahlskog JE, Muenter MD: **Frequency of levodopa-related dyskinesias and motor fluctuations as estimated from the cumulative literature.** *Mov Disord* 2001, **16**(3):448-458.
7. Kieburtz K: **Therapeutic strategies to prevent motor complications in Parkinson's disease.** *J Neurol* 2008, **255 Suppl 4**:42-45.
8. Ecker D, Unrath A, Kassubek J, Sabolek M: **Dopamine Agonists and their risk to induce psychotic episodes in Parkinson's disease: a case-control study.** *BMC Neurol* 2009, **9**:23.
9. Antonini A, Tolosa E, Mizuno Y, Yamamoto M, Poewe WH: **A reassessment of risks and benefits of dopamine agonists in Parkinson's disease.** *Lancet Neurol* 2009, **8**(10):929-937.
10. Lindvall O, Hagell P: **Cell therapy and transplantation in Parkinson's disease.** *Clin Chem Lab Med* 2001, **39**(4):356-361.
11. Lindvall O, Hagell P: **Role of cell therapy in Parkinson disease.** *Neurosurgical focus* 2002, **13**(5):e2.
12. Lindvall O, Bjorklund A: **Cell therapy in Parkinson's disease.** *NeuroRx* 2004, **1**(4):382-393.
13. Olanow CW, Goetz CG, Kordower JH, Stoessl AJ, Sossi V, Brin MF, Shannon KM, Nauert GM, Perl DP, Godbold J et al: **A double-blind controlled trial of bilateral fetal nigral transplantation in Parkinson's disease.** *Annals of neurology* 2003, **54**(3):403-414.
14. Mendez I, Vinuela A, Astradsson A, Mukhida K, Hallett P, Robertson H, Tierney T, Holness R, Dagher A, Trojanowski JQ et al: **Dopamine neurons implanted into people with Parkinson's disease survive without pathology for 14 years.** *Nature medicine* 2008, **14**(5):507-509.
15. Buddensiek J, Dressel A, Kowalski M, Storch A, Sabolek M: **Adult cerebrospinal fluid inhibits neurogenesis but facilitates gliogenesis from fetal rat neural stem cells.** *Journal of neuroscience research* 2009, **87**(14):3054-3066.
16. Blum B, Benvenisty N: **The tumorigenicity of human embryonic stem cells.** *Adv Cancer Res* 2008, **100**:133-158.
17. Doss MX, Koehler CI, Gissel C, Hescheler J, Sachinidis A: **Embryonic stem cells: a promising tool for cell replacement therapy.** *Journal of cellular and molecular medicine* 2004, **8**(4):465-473.

18. Przyborski SA: **Differentiation of human embryonic stem cells after transplantation in immune-deficient mice.** *Stem cells (Dayton, Ohio)* 2005, **23**(9):1242-1250.
19. Baker DE, Harrison NJ, Maltby E, Smith K, Moore HD, Shaw PJ, Heath PR, Holden H, Andrews PW: **Adaptation to culture of human embryonic stem cells and oncogenesis in vivo.** *Nature biotechnology* 2007, **25**(2):207-215.
20. Harris DT, Badowski M, Ahmad N, Gaballa MA: **The potential of cord blood stem cells for use in regenerative medicine.** *Expert opinion on biological therapy* 2007, **7**(9):1311-1322.
21. Hermann A, Gastl R, Liebau S, Popa MO, Fiedler J, Boehm BO, Maisel M, Lerche H, Schwarz J, Brenner R *et al*: **Efficient generation of neural stem cell-like cells from adult human bone marrow stromal cells.** *Journal of cell science* 2004, **117**(Pt 19):4411-4422.
22. Hermann A, Maisel M, Storch A: **Epigenetic conversion of human adult bone mesodermal stromal cells into neuroectodermal cell types for replacement therapy of neurodegenerative disorders.** *Expert opinion on biological therapy* 2006, **6**(7):653-670.
23. Parker AM, Katz AJ: **Adipose-derived stem cells for the regeneration of damaged tissues.** *Expert opinion on biological therapy* 2006, **6**(6):567-578.
24. Vogel W, Grunebach F, Messam CA, Kanz L, Brugger W, Buhring HJ: **Heterogeneity among human bone marrow-derived mesenchymal stem cells and neural progenitor cells.** *Haematologica* 2003, **88**(2):126-133.
25. Uchida N, Buck DW, He D, Reitsma MJ, Masek M, Phan TV, Tsukamoto AS, Gage FH, Weissman IL: **Direct isolation of human central nervous system stem cells.** *Proceedings of the National Academy of Sciences of the United States of America* 2000, **97**(26):14720-14725.
26. Aubert J, Stavridis MP, Tweedie S, O'Reilly M, Vierlinger K, Li M, Ghazal P, Pratt T, Mason JO, Roy D *et al*: **Screening for mammalian neural genes via fluorescence-activated cell sorter purification of neural precursors from Sox1-gfp knock-in mice.** *Proceedings of the National Academy of Sciences of the United States of America* 2003, **100 Suppl 1**:11836-11841.
27. Watson MA, Scott MG: **Clinical utility of biochemical analysis of cerebrospinal fluid.** *Clin Chem* 1995, **41**(3):343-360.
28. Buddensiek J, Dressel A, Kowalski M, Runge U, Schroeder H, Hermann A, Kirsch M, Storch A, Sabolek M: **Cerebrospinal fluid promotes survival and astroglial differentiation of adult human neural progenitor cells but inhibits proliferation and neuronal differentiation.** *BMC neuroscience*, **11**(1):48.
29. Kordower JH, Chu Y, Hauser RA, Freeman TB, Olanow CW: **Lewy body-like pathology in long-term embryonic nigral transplants in Parkinson's disease.** *Nature medicine* 2008, **14**(5):504-506.
30. Li JY, Englund E, Holton JL, Soulet D, Hagell P, Lees AJ, Lashley T, Quinn NP, Rehncrona S, Bjorklund A *et al*: **Lewy bodies in grafted neurons in subjects with Parkinson's disease suggest host-to-graft disease propagation.** *Nature medicine* 2008, **14**(5):501-503.
31. Kordower JH, Chu Y, Hauser RA, Olanow CW, Freeman TB: **Transplanted dopaminergic neurons develop PD pathologic changes: a second case report.** *Mov Disord* 2008, **23**(16):2303-2306.
32. Cicchetti F, Saporta S, Hauser RA, Parent M, Saint-Pierre M, Sanberg PR, Li XJ, Parker JR, Chu Y, Mufson EJ *et al*: **Neural transplants in patients with Huntington's disease undergo disease-like neuronal degeneration.** *Proceedings of the National Academy of Sciences of the United States of America* 2009, **106**(30):12483-12488.

33. Brundin P, Li JY, Holton JL, Lindvall O, Revesz T: **Research in motion: the enigma of Parkinson's disease pathology spread**. *Nat Rev Neurosci* 2008, **9**(10):741-745.
34. Lindvall O, Kokaia Z, Martinez-Serrano A: **Stem cell therapy for human neurodegenerative disorders-how to make it work**. *Nature medicine* 2004, **10 Suppl**:S42-50.
35. Andres RH, Meyer M, Ducray AD, Widmer HR: **Restorative neuroscience: concepts and perspectives**. *Swiss Med Wkly* 2008, **138**(11-12):155-172.
36. Ren Z, Zhang Y: **Cells therapy for Parkinson's disease--so close and so far away**. *Sci China C Life Sci* 2009, **52**(7):610-614.
37. Hermann A, Storch A: **Endogenous regeneration in Parkinson's disease: do we need orthotopic dopaminergic neurogenesis?** *Stem cells (Dayton, Ohio)* 2008, **26**(11):2749-2752.
38. Geraerts M, Krylyshkina O, Debyser Z, Baekelandt V: **Concise review: therapeutic strategies for Parkinson disease based on the modulation of adult neurogenesis**. *Stem cells (Dayton, Ohio)* 2007, **25**(2):263-270.
39. Weaver FM, Follett K, Stern M, Hur K, Harris C, Marks WJ, Jr., Rothlind J, Sagher O, Reda D, Moy CS *et al*: **Bilateral deep brain stimulation vs best medical therapy for patients with advanced Parkinson disease: a randomized controlled trial**. *JAMA* 2009, **301**(1):63-73.
40. Lindvall O, Kokaia Z: **Stem cells for the treatment of neurological disorders**. *Nature* 2006, **441**(7097):1094-1096.

7. Appendices

7.1 Acknowledgements

I wish to thank Dr. Michael Sabolek for the very amicable support during the years of these experiments. Especially I want to thank him for the "always open door" policy he gave and for his enthusiasm for neuroscience, which has infected me. I am truly grateful for all the opportunities I had to attend international congresses and to gain experiences in presenting posters, writing papers and giving lectures.

Sigrid Peters I want to acknowledge for expert technical assistance, for having an ear for all smaller and larger problems during my time in the laboratory and for being more than helpful whenever she could.

I would like to thank Prof. Dr. Henry Schroeder and Prof. Dr. Uwe Runge for providing the human brain tissue and PD. Dr. Alexander Dressel for the supply and inspection of human adult CSF samples.

Furthermore I would like to acknowledge the Department of Surgery for the permission to use their fluorescence microscope and the Department of Transfusion medicine for making it possible to use their LightCylcler System for RT-PCR Analysis.

Prof. Dr. med. Dr. h.c. Christof Kessler I wish to thank for being my Ph.D. supervisor and for making it possible to conduct all my experiments in his clinic.

I am truly grateful to Prof. Dr. Alexander Storch and Dr. Andreas Hermann for helping with some of the immunostainings, for reading and correcting paper manuscript and for being helpful advisors for all larger problems we had in the laboratory.

Hendrik and Trudie I would like to thank for helping with the layout and revising the manuscript of my Ph.D. thesis.

Last but not least I'm most grateful to my parents for supporting me in every possible way during all the years as well as to the rest of my family and my fiancé for all their help, patience and interest.

7.2 Referred publications

Buddensiek J, Dressel A, Kowalski M, Storch A, Sabolek M: Adult cerebrospinal fluid inhibits neurogenesis but facilitates gliogenesis from fetal rat neural stem cells. *Journal of neuroscience research* 2009, 87(14):3054-3066.

Buddensiek J, Dressel A, Kowalski M, Runge U, Schroeder H, Hermann A, Kirsch M, Storch A, Sabolek M: Cerebrospinal fluid promotes survival and astroglial differentiation of adult human neural progenitor cells but inhibits proliferation and neuronal differentiation. *BMC neuroscience*, 11(1):48.

Adult Cerebrospinal Fluid Inhibits Neurogenesis but Facilitates Gliogenesis from Fetal Rat Neural Stem Cells

Judith Buddensiek,[1] Alexander Dressel,[1] Michael Kowalski,[1] Alexander Storch,[2] and Michael Sabolek[1]*

[1]Department of Neurology, EMA University of Greifswald, Greifswald, Germany
[2]Department of Neurology and Center for Regenerative Therapies Dresden (CRTD), Dresden University of Technology, Dresden, Germany

Neural stem cells (NSCs) are a promising source for cell replacement therapies for neurological diseases. Administration of NSCs into the cerebrospinal fluid (CSF) offers a nontraumatic transplantation method into the brain. However, cell survival and intraparenchymal migration of the transplants are limited. Furthermore, CSF was recently reported to be an important milieu for controlling stem cell processes in the brain. We studied the effects of adult human leptomeningeal CSF on the behavior of fetal rat NSCs. CSF increased survival of NSCs compared with standard culture media during stem cell maintenance and differentiation. The presence of CSF enhanced NSC differentiation, leading to a faster loss of self-renewal capacity and faster and stronger neurite outgrowth. Some of these effects (mainly cell survival, neurite brancing) were blocked by addition of the bone morphogenic protein (BMP) inhibitor noggin. After differentiation in CSF, significantly fewer MAP2ab$^+$ neurons were found, but there were more GFAP$^+$ astroglia compared with standard media. By RT-PCR analysis, we determined a decrease of mRNA of the NSC marker gene *Nestin* but an increase of *Gfap* mRNA during differentiation up to 72 hr in CSF compared with standard media. Our data demonstrate that adult human leptomeningeal CSF enhances cell survival of fetal rat NSCs during proliferation and differentiation. Furthermore, CSF provides a stimulus for gliogenesis but inhibits neurogenesis from fetal NSCs. Our data suggest that CSF contains factors such as BMPs regulating NSC behavior, and we hypothesize that fast differentiation of NSCs in CSF leads to a rapid loss of migration capacity of intrathecally transplanted NSCs. © 2009 Wiley-Liss, Inc.

Key words: cerebrospinal fluid (CSF); neural stem cells; neural differentiation

Neural stem cells (NSCs) are a promising source for cell replacement therapies in the brain (Sievertzon et al., 2005). They can be extracted from fetal CNS (McKay, 1997; Svendsen et al., 1999; Gage, 2000) or generated by embryonal stem cells (ESCs; Bain et al., 1995; Gage, 2000; Kawasaki et al., 2000, 2002; Lee et al., 2000). Furthermore, NSCs can be isolated from different regions of the adult brain, such as the hippocampus and the subventricular zone (SVZ) of the lateral ventricles, and from some nonneurogenic regions (Reynolds and Weiss, 1992; McKay, 1997; Johansson et al., 1999; Gage, 2000; Magavi et al., 2000; Shihabuddin et al., 2000; Rietze et al., 2001). As derivatives of the neuroectodermal tissue, NSCs are able to generate all cell types of nervous tissue, such as neurons, astroglia, and oligodendroglia (McKay, 1997; Gage, 2000; Storch et al., 2004). Several promising candidates as markers for NSCs, such as nestin and musashi, turned out to be unreliable because they were also expressed in non-NSCs (Cai et al., 2003). During in vitro expansion, NSCs grow in multicellular aggregates, so-called neurospheres, or under adherent conditions (Reynolds and Weiss, 1992; McKay, 1997; Johansson et al., 1999; Storch et al., 2001, 2004). The removal of the mitogens EGF/FGF leads to spontaneous differentiation of NSCs. As we previously reported, under the conditions described, NSCs from rodent fetal midbrain differentiate primarily into astroglia (37%) and to a lesser extent into oligodendrocytes (13%) and neurons (23%; Sabolek et al., 2006).

In vivo analyses of intrastriatally transplanted cultured rodent and human adult and fetal NSCs show long-term survival, extensive distribution, and morphological maturation in rats (Svendsen et al., 1997; Fricker et al., 1999; Jain et al., 2006; Lepore et al., 2006; Vazey

Contract grant sponsor: Department Neurowissenschaften der der Ernst-Moritz-Arndt University of Greifswald (to J.B., M.S.); Contract grant sponsor: Konrad Adenauer Stiftung (to J.B.).

*Correspondence to: Michael Sabolek, Department of Neurology, EMA University of Greifswald, Sauerbruchstrasse, 17489 Greifswald, Germany. E-mail: michael.sabolek@uni-greifswald.de

Received 21 January 2009; Revised 16 April 2009; Accepted 7 May 2009

Published online 15 June 2009 in Wiley InterScience (www.interscience.wiley.com). DOI: 10.1002/jnr.22150

© 2009 Wiley-Liss, Inc.

et al., 2006; Olstorn et al., 2007; Darsalia et al., 2007). Transplanted NSCs also formed synapses, suggesting integration into adult rodent CNS (Lepore et al., 2006). It has also been reported that transplantation of NSCs leads to a reduction of functional impairment in animal models of different neurodegenerative disorders such as Huntington' s disease (Vazey et al., 2006), Parkinson's disease (Kitayama et al., 2007; Wei et al., 2007), and amyotrophic lateral sclerosis (ALS; Corti et al., 2007; Martin and Liu, 2007) and in animal stroke models (Jeong et al., 2003; Chu et al., 2004; Lee et al., 2007). So far, NSCs have been transplanted predominantly directly into the rodent CNS (Svendsen et al., 1997; Fricker et al., 1999; Jain et al., 2006; Lepore et al., 2006; Vazey et al., 2006; Corti et al., 2007; Darsalia et al., 2007; Kitayama et al., 2007; Lee et al., 2007; Martin and Liu, 2007; Olstorn et al., 2007; Wei et al., 2007), but, in recent reports, nontraumatic transplantation into the CNS via cerebrospinal fluid (CSF) has been demonstrated. In different studies, an intensive invasion, migration, and integration of transplanted NSCs into the damaged CNS have been detected after transplantation via CSF (Wu et al., 2002a,b; Bai et al., 2003; Ohta et al., 2004). In a very recent report, intrathecal application of neuroectodermally converted human bone marrow-derived mesodermal stromal cells (hMSC-NSCs) in the cisterna magna of an ALS mouse model has been reported (Habisch et al., 2007). Interestingly, the transplanted cells did not migrate into the CNS in sufficient amounts to prolong the survival of transgenic ALS mice or to delay the first signs of disease. As a possible reason, a low survival rate of intrathecally applied cells resulting from the low nutrient content of the CSF was discussed (Habisch et al., 2007).

Growing evidence suggests that CSF plays an important role not only in brain development but also in survival, proliferation, and differentiation of neuroectodermal stem cells (Mashayekhi et al., 2002; Gato et al., 2004, 2005; Martin et al., 2006; Johanson et al., 2008; Bachy et al., 2008). How CSF influences neuroectodermal cells during development remains, however, enigmatic, but the components contained in CSF as well as CSF pressure and flow seem to play an important role (Johanson et al., 2008). Regarding the components of CSF influencing neuroectodermal cells, recent investigations concentrated mainly on proteins, "membranous particles," and amino acids but also on growth factors such as FGF2 (Parada et al., 2005; Martin et al., 2006; Nordin et al., 2007; Bachy et al., 2008). Most investigations concerning the influence of CSF contents on survival, proliferation, and differentiation are performed with embryonic avian CSF (Gato et al., 2004, 2005; Bachy et al., 2008), but there are well-known differences between avian and mammalian CSF (Parada et al., 2005). Because no studies using human CSF have been published yet, the effects of human CSF on neural stem or progenitors cells are unclear. We therefore tested here the effects of human adult CSF on the in vitro behavior of fetal rat midbrain NSCs.

MATERIALS AND METHODS

Collection of Adult Human Leptomeningeal CSF

The CSF samples were taken for diagnostic purpose from adult patients in the Neurological Clinic of the Ernst Moritz Arndt University of Greifswald by a lumbar puncture. All patients gave a written informed consent for the diagnostic procedure. Lumbar puncture was performed by standard protocols. The final diagnosis for all patients whose CSF was used was idiopathic normal pressure hydrocephalus (NPH). In all patients, tumors and infectious diseases were excluded. Surplus CSF from diagnostic samples of all patients was spun down to remove remaining cells, pooled, and analyzed to exclude nonsterility and presence of inflammatory markers. The pooled CSF was normal in all standard parameters, and contamination with blood was excluded. The exact parameters were as follows: cell count $<1/\mu l$, no blood contamination, normal protein of 369 mg/liter, normal glucose of 3.6 mmol/liter, normal lactate of 2.0 mmol/liter, normal ferritin of 7.2 µg/liter, normal albumin quotient of 5.0×10^{-3}, normal immunoglobulin quotients of IgG 2.1×10^{-3}, IgA 1.1×10^{-3}, IgM $<0.2 \times 10^{-3}$. Scientific use of CSF samples was approved by the local Ethics Committee. Pooled CSF samples were aliquoted and frozen at $-80°C$ until use.

Isolation and Propagation of Fetal Rat NSCs

Mesencephalic NSCs from E14.5 rat embryonic brain were prepared as previously described (Storch et al., 2003; Milosevic et al., 2004). In brief, pregnant females (Wistar rats; Charles River, Braunschweig, Germany) were sacrificed according to NIH guidelines. For expansion of neurospheres, tissue samples were dissociated using trypsin, DNase, and mechanical trituration. The cells were added to 25-cm^2 flasks and maintained in serum-free media comprising DMEM/F-12 mixture (2:1) supplemented with 2% B27 supplement, 2% penicillin/streptomycin, and 20 ng/ml EGF. Cultures were incubated at 37°C in a humidified atmosphere and lowered O_2 conditions of 5% CO_2, 92% N_2, and 3% ± 2% O_2. Fresh medium and growth factors were supplemented every 5 days. For bromodeoxyuridine (BrdU) labelling, cells were incubated with 10 µm BrdU for 24 hr. Some of the expansion experiments were conducted in the presence of 150 ng/ml noggin, a bone morphogenic protein (BMP) inhibitor. Cells were used between passage 3 and passage 11 for experiments to avoid contamination with primary cells. The NSCs used grow as long-term expanded "neurosphere" cultures in a well-defined and homogenous system expressing the stem cell marker nestin in 86.7% ± 5.7% (n = 3) of the cells not expressing GFAP or Tuj1. The early neuronal marker Tuj1 is present in only a small proportion of cells (4.2% ± 0.7%), a small subfraction also being positive for nestin (0.6% ± 0.3%), indicating that the nestin$^+$ neuronal precursor population was undergoing spontaneous differentiation in culture. The astrocyte marker GFAP was present in only a small fraction of cells, and only 2.1% ± 0.8% of cells were positive for both nestin and GFAP (data not shown).

TABLE I. Primers for Semiquantitative Real-Time RT-PCR

Gene (protein)	Sequence (forward, reverse)	Product length (bp)	Accession No.
Gfap(GFAP)	5'-GGT ATC GGT CCA AGT TTG C-3' 5'-GCC TCT CCA AGG ACT CGT TC-3'	159	NM_017009
Hmbs (hydroxymethylbilane synthase)	5'-TGT ATG CTG TGG GTC AGG GAG-3' 5'-CTC CTT CCA GGT GCC TCA GA-3'	144	NM_013168
Nes (nestin)	5'-CAC TGA TAA GTT CCA GCT GGC-3' 5'-CAG AGT CCT GTA TGT AGC CAC C-3'	148	NM_012987
Tubb3 (β-tubulin class III)	5'-GCC TCC TCT CAC AAG TAT G-3' 5'-CAG CAC CAC TCT GAC CGA AG-3'	133	NM_139254

Differentiation Conditions

Cells were differentiated by plating them onto poly-L-lysine-coated chamber slides or six-well plates in P4-8F with 2% penicillin/streptomycin (standard serum-free cell culture media; from AthenaES, Baltimore, MD) without addition of any growth factors or serum supplement or in CSF, respectively. Notably, the albumin content of P4-8F of 250 μg/ml matches the normal albumin content of healthy adult lumbar CSF. Also, the glucose content of P4-8F is in a physiological concentration of 7 mmol/liter. The cells were allowed to differentiate for 10–14 days at 37°C in a humidified atmosphere at lowered O_2 conditions of 5% CO_2, 92% N_2, and 3% ± 2% O_2. Half of the media was changed every third day. Some of the differentiation experiments were conducted in the presence of 150 ng/ml recombinant noggin (R&D System, Minneapolis, MN). For investigating cell morphology, survival rate, and marker expression by immunocytochemistry, the cultures were fixed from 0 up to 72 hr and 14 days after starting the differentiation process. For analyses of gene expression on mRNA, cells were harvested at 0, 3, 6, and 72 hr after initiation of differentiation.

Immunostainings

For immunocytochemistry, cell cultures were fixed in 4% paraformaldehyde in PBS or with 4% paraformaldehyde/PBS, followed by ice-cold acidic ethanol and 2 N HCl for BrdU staining. Immuncytochemistry was carried out by using standard protocols. Cell nuclei were counterstained with 4,6-diamidino-2-phenylindole (DAPI). To determine the self-renewing potential of NSCs, Ki67 and BrdU incorporation was used. Ki67 is detected in the nucleus of proliferating cells in all active phases of the cell cycle from the late G1 phase though the M phase (Gerdes et al., 1983, 1984). BrdU marks cells within the S phase of the cell cycle (Eisch and Mandyam, 2007). Antibodies and dilutions were as follows: rabbit antiglial fibrillary acidic protein (GFAP) polyclonal 1:1,000 (Chemicon International, Temecula, CA), mouse anti-MAP2 monoclonal 1:100 (Pharmingen, San Diego, CA), mouse antigalactocerebroside monoclonal 1:500 (Chemicon), rabbit anti-Ki67 polyclonal 1:500 (Berlin Chemie AG, Berlin, Germany), mouse anti-BrdU 1:16 (Roche Applied Science, Mannheim, Germany), and secondary antibodies conjugated to Alexa 488 and 594 1:500 (Gibco/Invitrogen, Carlsbad, CA).

For determining the survival rate during expansion and differentiation, dead cells were stained with propidium iodide 1:50 (Sigma Aldrich, St. Louis, MO), and cell nuclei were counterstained with Hoechst 33342 1:1,000 (Sigma Aldrich). Images were captured with an inverse fluorescence microscope (Inversionsmikroskop Leica DMIL; Leica, Wetzlar, Germany).

Cell Counts, Measurements of Neurites, and Statistical Analysis

For quantification of the percentage of cells expressing a given marker, the number of positive cells of at least five representative areas per experiment was determined relative to the total number of DAPI/Hoechst-labelled nuclei. In a typical experiment, in total 500–1,000 cells were counted per marker. The mean values for more than three conditions are given together with SDs. Statistical comparisons were made by ANOVA with post hoc t-test or Dunnett's t-test where appropriate. All data are presented as mean ± SEM. $P < 0.05$ was considered statistically significant.

RNA Extraction and Quantitative RT-PCR Analysis

RNA extraction and semiquantitative RT-PCR were performed as described previously (Hermann et al., 2004). In brief, total cellular RNA was extracted from NPCs using an RNAeasy mini kit (Qiagen, Valencia, CA), following the manufacturer's recommendations. Semiquantitative real-time one-step RT-PCR was carried out with the LightCycler System (Roche), and amplification was monitored and analyzed by measuring the binding of the fluorescence dye SYBR Green I to double-stranded DNA. One microliter (50 ng) of total RNA was reverse transcribed and subsequently amplified with QuantiTect SYBR Green RT-PCR Master mix (Qiagen) and 0.5 μmol/liter^{-1} of both sense and antisense primers. Tenfold dilutions of total RNA were used as external standards. Standards and samples were simultaneously amplified. After amplification, melting curves of the RT-PCR products were acquired to demonstrate product specificity. The results are expressed relative to the housekeeping gene Hmbs (hydroxymethylbilane synthase). The relative RNA content was determined by using the formula of the comparative cycle threshold (Ct): TG/RG = 2Ct(RG) − Ct(TG) (Livak and Schmittgen, 2001). Primer sequences, lengths of the amplified products, and melting point analyses are summarized in Table I.

RESULTS

CSF Increases the Survival Rate of Fetal Rat NSCs

After in vitro expansion for at least three passages in standard media, NSCs were transferred to uncoated chamber slides and expanded in standard expansion medium or CSF with or without 150 ng/ml noggin for an additional 72 hr. Thereafter, cells were stained with Hoechst 33342 and propidium iodide to determine the amount of dead cells. Our results showed a significantly higher survival rate of NSCs in CSF compared with expansion medium (see Materials and Methods), with 16.0% ± 1.2% of dead cells in expansion medium vs. 1.9% ± 0.6% of dead cells in CSF. Addition of noggin completely blocked the CSF effects (15.2% ± 6.8% necrotic cells; Fig. 1). Similar results were obtained after differentiating the cells in standard media (P4-8F) or CSF with or without 150 ng/ml noggin on PLL-coated chamber slides for 24 and 72 hr, with significantly higher survival rates in CSF compared with P4-8F media and inhibition of this CSF effect by addition of noggin. In P4-8F, 34.8% ± 20.5% of NSCs were found dead 24 hr after the beginning of differentiation, but only 3.3% ± 1.1% of NSCs showed cell death in CSF without noggin (Fig. 2). Addition of noggin increased cell death rates to those of control conditions with 22.5% ± 7.3% of dead NSCs. After 72 hr, 13.3% ± 5.7% and 2.5% ± 1.1% of NSCs were found dead in P4-8F and CSF, respectively (Fig. 2).

CSF Inhibits NSC Proliferation

To determine the proliferation potential of the investigated NSCs, we used the proliferation marker Ki67 as well as BrdU incorporation. After in vitro expansion of at least three passages, the cells were transferred to uncoated chamber slides and expanded in culture medium or CSF with or without 150 ng/ml noggin. The proliferation parameters were determined at 24 or 72 hr after changing the media. At each investigated time point, the percentages of Ki67$^+$ and BrdU$^+$ NSCs were significantly higher in expansion medium compared with those in CSF, representing a larger number of cells with proliferation potential. Hence, after 24 hr, 30.2% ± 0.6% of NSCs were BrdU$^+$ in expansion media vs. 20.1% ± 1.3% in CSF. After 72 hr, Ki67 was detected in 2.4% ± 1.4% of NSCs expanded in expansion media and 0.4% ± 0.3% of NSCs expanded in CSF. Addition of noggin did not reverse the CSF effects observed with BrdU staining (20.4% ± 2.2% BrdU$^+$ cells) but only on Ki67 staining (1.6% ± 0.4%; Fig. 3).

CSF Increases Extension Outgrowth Velocity From NSCs

We used the time course of extension outgrowth as a first measure of the differentiation process of NSCs in cultures. Thus, after in vitro expansion for at least three passages, NSCs were allowed to differentiate. They were plated onto PLL-coated chamber slides in either P4-8F media or CSF with or without 150 ng/ml noggin. For investigating extension outgrowth, number and length of extensions were determined at 0, 3, 6, 24, and 72 hr after starting the differentiation process. Comparing results in P4-8F and CSF, the difference was most striking during the first 6 hr with longer neurites in CSF

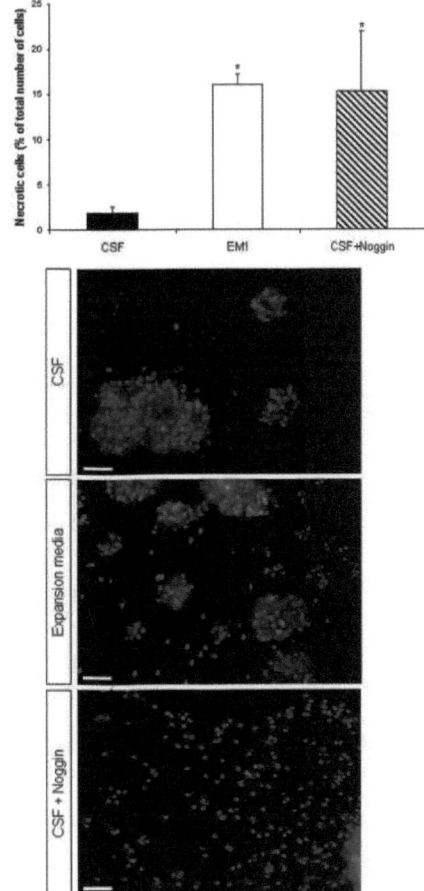

Fig. 1. Survival rates of NSCs during expansion. **A:** Percentage of necrotic NSCs expanded in standard expansion media or CSF with or without 150 ng/ml of noggin for 72 hr. Values represent the mean ± SEM from at least three independent experiments. *$P <$ 0.05. **B:** Representative microphotographs demonstrating the influence of CSF on survival rate of NSCs. For immunostainings, dead cells were stained with propidium iodide. Nuclei were counterstained with Hoechst 33342. The upper panel shows NSCs expanded in CSF, the middle panel shows NSCs expanded in expansion media supplemented with EGF, and the lower panel shows NSCs expanded in CSF + noggin. Scale bars = 50 μm. [Color figure can be viewed in the online issue, which is available at www.interscience.wiley.com.]

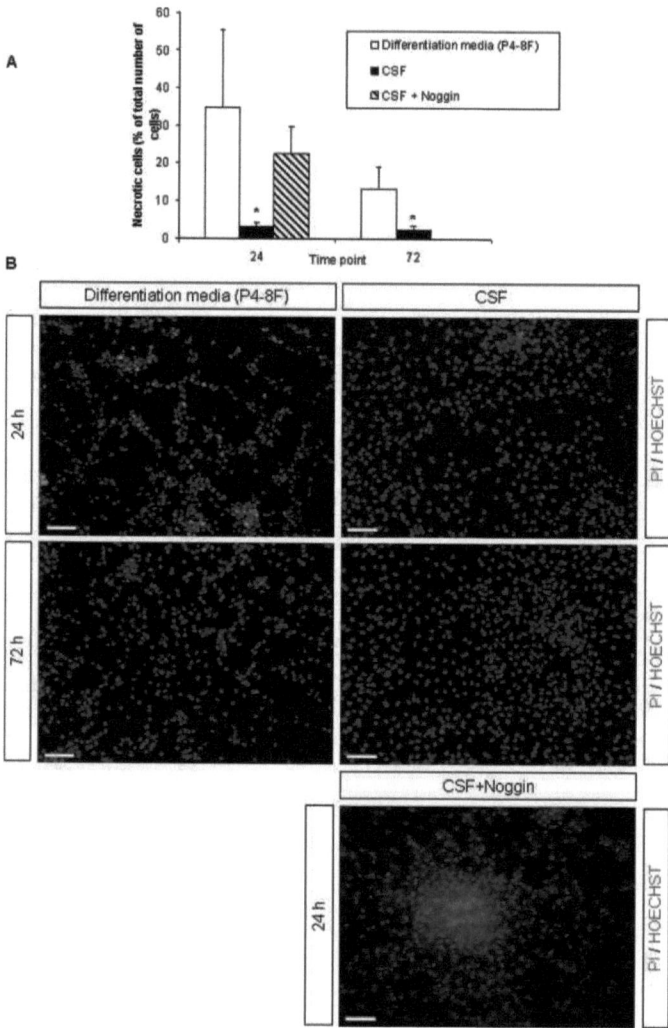

Fig. 2. Survival rates of NSCs during differentiation. **A:** The percentage of necrotic NSCs at 24 and 72 hr after differentiation on PLL-coated chamber slides in standard differentiation media (P4-8F) or CSF with or without 150 ng/ml noggin. Values represent the mean ± SEM from at least three independent experiments. *$P < 0.05$. **B:** Representative microphotographs demonstrating the influence of CSF on the survival rate of NSCs. For immunostainings, dead cells were stained with propidium iodide. Nuclei were counterstained with Hoechst 33342. Scale bars = 50 µm. [Color figure can be viewed in the online issue, which is available at www.interscience.wiley.com.]

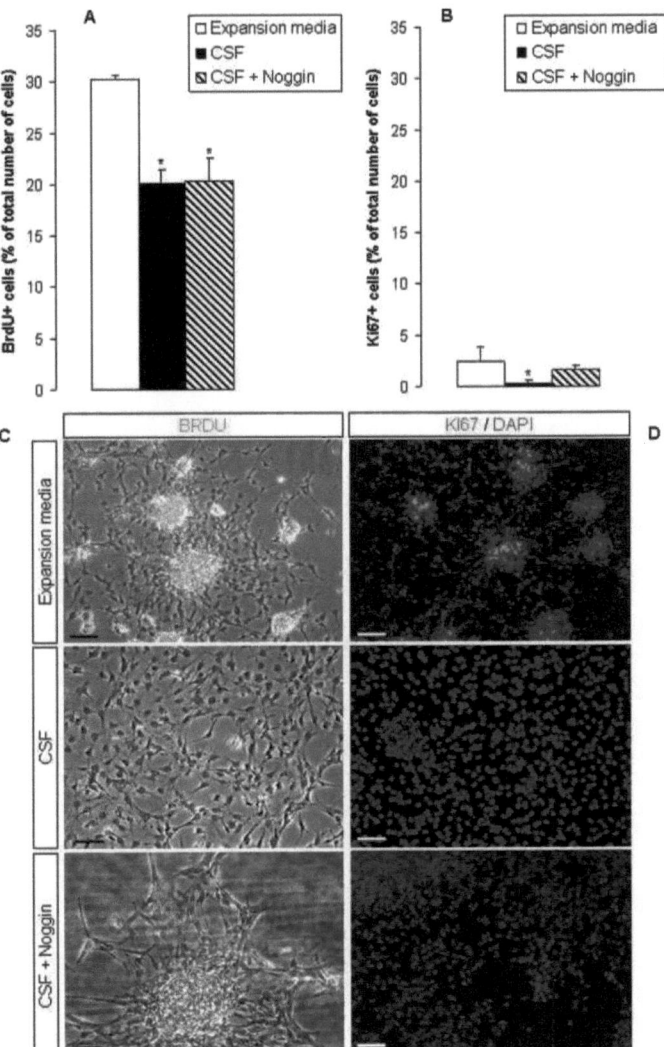

Fig. 3. Proliferation potential of NSCs during expansion. **A,B:** The percentage of NSCs with potential to self-renewal expanded in standard expansion media or in CSF with or without 150 ng/ml noggin after 24 (A: anti-BrdU) and 72 (B: Anti-Ki67) hr. Values represent the mean ± SEM from at least three independent experiments. *$P <$ 0.05. **C,D:** Representative microphotographs demonstrating the influence of CSF on proliferation potential of NSCs. For immunolabelling, cells were stained with anti-BrdU (C) and anti-Ki67 (D). Nuclei were counterstained with DAPI (D). C: NSCs expanded in expansion media (upper panel)/CSF (middle panel)/CSF + noggin (lower panel) for 24 hr. D: NSCs expanded in expansion media (upper panel)/CSF (middle panel)/CSF + noggin (lower panel) for 72 hr. Scale bars = 50 μm. [Color figure can be viewed in the online issue, which is available at www.interscience.wiley.com.]

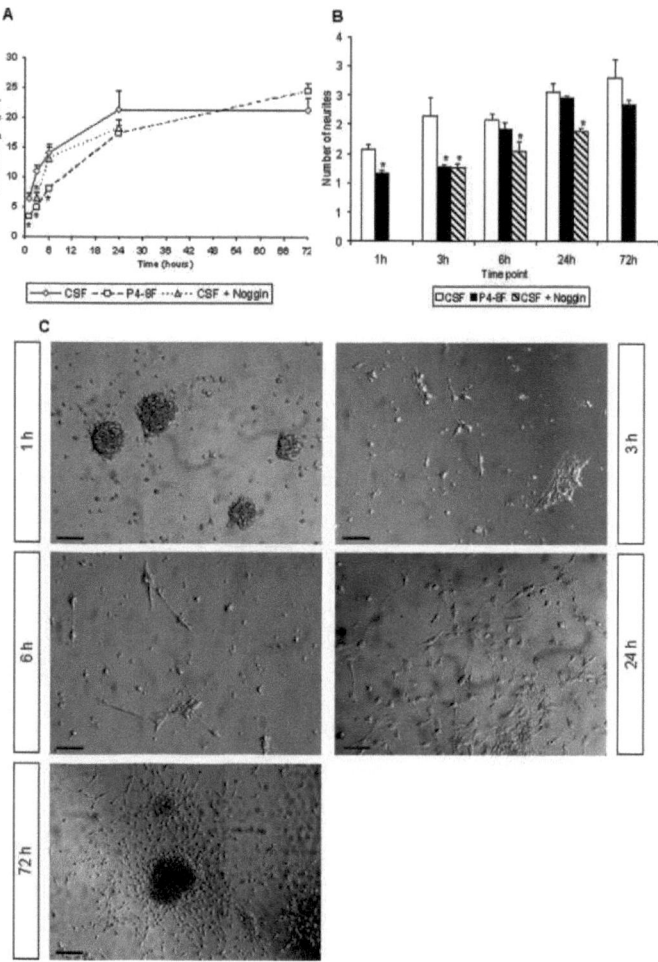

Fig. 4. Extension outgrowth from NSCs. **A:** Neurite length (in μm) after 0, 3, 6, 24, and 72 hr of differentiation in standard media (P4-8F) or CSF with or without 150 ng/ml noggin. **B:** Number of neurites at 0, 3, 6, 24, and 72 hr of differentiation in P4-8F or CSF with or without 150 ng/ml noggin. Values represent the mean ± SEM from at least three independent experiments. *$P < 0.05$ (post hoc t-test). **C:** Representative microphotographs showing the morphology of NSCs at 0, 3, 6, 24, and 72 hr of differentiation in CSF. Scale bars = 50 μm. [Color figure can be viewed in the online issue, which is available at www.interscience.wiley.com.]

($P < 0.0001$; F-value: 38.746, ANOVA), whereas final neurite length did not differ significantly. Addition of noggin only inhibited the CSF effects at 3 hr. A significantly larger number of neurites could be determined in CSF only during the first 3 hr of differentiation ($P < 0.0001$; F-value: 17.716, ANOVA; Fig. 4). Addition of noggin to CSF led to a significantly smaller number of neurites at the observed time points 3, 6, and 24 hr, which was even smaller than in P4-8F.

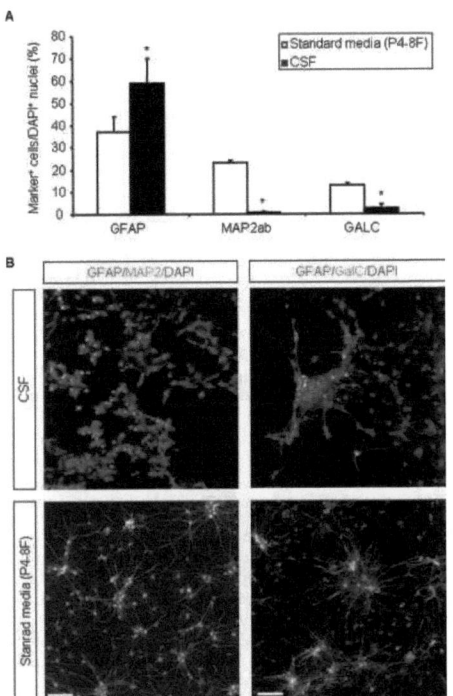

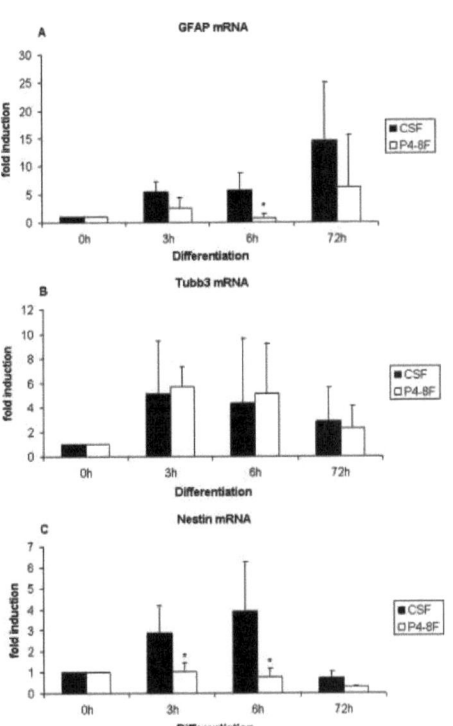

Fig. 5. Gliogenesis and neurogenesis from NSCs. **A:** Quantitative data for GFAP, MAP2ab, and GALC expression obtained by triple stainings of NSCs, differentiated for 10–14 days in P48F/CSF. Medium/CSF was changed every 3 days. Results are mean values ± SEM from at least three independent experiments. *$P < 0.05$. **B:** Representative microphotographs demonstrating the effects of CSF on neuronal and glial differentiation of NSCs 10–14 days after initiation of the differentiation process. Cells were stained for GFAP/MAP2 and GalC. Nuclei were counterstained with DAPI. Scale bar = 50 μm. [Color figure can be viewed in the online issue, which is available at www.interscience.wiley.com.]

Fig. 6. Gene expression pattern during differentiation of NSCs. Gene expression relative to the housekeeping gene *Hmbs* by RT-PCR. **A:** *Gfap*. **B:** *Tubb3*. **C:** *Nestin*. Differentiation period were 1, 3, 6, and 72 hr. Values represent the mean ± SEM from at least three independent experiments. *$P < 0.05$.

CSF Inhibits Neurogenesis but Activates Gliogenesis From NSCs

We recently demonstrated that 37% ± 7% of midbrain NSCs plated in P4-8F onto PLL-coated chamber slides differentiate into GFAP$^+$ astroglia, 13% ± 1% into galactocerebrosidase (GalC)$^+$ oligodendrocytes, and 23% ± 1% into microtubule-associated protein 2 (MAP2)$^+$ neurons (Sabolek et al., 2006). To elucidate the question of whether the presence of CSF influences gliogenesis, oligodendrogenesis, or neurogenesis, NSCs were allowed to differentiate for 10–14 days on PLL-coated chamber slides in either P4-8F or CSF. After 10–14 days of differentiation in CSF, the distribution of mature neuroectodermal cell populations was significantly different compared with that in standard media. In CSF, 58.9% ± 12.1% of NSCs acquired phenotypic characteristics of astrocytes (GFAP$^+$), 2.4% ± 2.5% those of oligodendrocytes (GalC$^+$), and 0.7% ± 0.6% those of mature neurons (MAP2$^+$; Fig. 5). In P4-8F, 47.0% ± 21.4% of NSCs acquired phenotypic characteristics of astrocytes (GFAP$^+$), 11.8% ± 2.5% those of oligodendrocytes (GalC$^+$), and 15.0% ± 2.8% those of mature neurons (MAP2$^+$; Fig. 5). Notably, the total amounts of cells expressing one of the three markers for mature neuroectodermal cell types were similar under both conditions (70.4% ± 12.7% and 64.3% ± 15.0% of DAPI-stained cells in P4-8F and CSF, respectively). Astroglial morphology differed in CSF and P4-8F, with smaller, less well arborized cells with rounder soma in CSF and cells with more complex arborization and thinner neurites in P4-8F (Fig. 5).

CSF Influences Gene Expression During Differentiation

To determine whether gene expression was influenced by CSF, gene expression analysis of neuroectodermal marker genes *Gfap*, *Nestin*, and *Tubb3* was carried out at 0, 3, 6, and 72 hr after starting the differentiation process using quantitative real-time RT-PCR. Our analyses showed a significant increase of *Nestin* mRNA 3 and 6 hr after starting the differentiation process in CSF compared with a gradual decrease of *Nestin* mRNA expression in P4-8F (Fig. 6A). After 72 hr, *Nestin* expression dropped significantly under the initial value in P4-8F. *Gfap* mRNA expression increased significantly at 6 hr after starting the differentiation process in CSF and continued to increase until the last examined time point, 72 hr. Also during differentiation in P4-8F, *Gfap* expression gradually increased over the whole observation period, but the increase was lower compared with differentiation in CSF for all examined time points, and the difference reached significance for the 6-hr time point. Also for *Tubb3* we found a parallel increase in mRNA expression for the first 6 hr of differentiation in CSF and P4-8F without a significant difference (Fig. 6C).

DISCUSSION

The central finding of our study is that, in vitro, adult human leptomeningeal CSF promotes survival and glial differentiation but inhibits neuronal specification of fetal NSCs compared with standard culture/differentiation conditions. Accordingly, the loss of stem cell potential of fetal NSCs is accelerated when cultured in CSF. These findings suggest that adult CSF contains key factors involved in the control of cellular proliferation and differentiation processes of fetal NSCs. Similar effects were reported for embryonic CSF, showing a trophic influence on survival, proliferation, and differentiation of neuroephitelial stem cells at early development stages. It has therefore already been postulated that diffusible factors in embryonic CSF regulate the three basic cellular behavioral parameters of neuroephitelial stem cells and that this CSF may play a key role in brain development in vivo (Gato et al., 2004, 2005; Parada et al., 2005; Martin et al., 2006; Bachy et al., 2008). Although it has been demonstrated that the protein composition of embryonic CSF is more complex than that of adult CSF (Gato et al., 2004), our results strongly suggest that adult CSF also has regulatory effects on stem cell behavior, for example, in the SVZ of the ventricular system. Indeed, adult NSCs of the SVZ have transitory contact with the ventricular brain cavities (Alvarez-Buylla and Garcia-Verdugo, 2002; Tramontin et al., 2003). In addition, our study provides potential explanations for the behavior of stem cells after transplantation into the CSF.

Fetal rat NSCs differentiated predominantly into astroglia, and only a very low amount of cells differentiated into neurons when exposed to CSF. Indeed, our data indicate that CSF further decreases the differentiation into neurons compared with standard serum-free differentiation media (Sabolek et al., 2006). Our findings are similar to those of previous studies showing astrogliogenesis after nontraumatic transplantation of NSCs via CSF (Bai et al., 2003). Neuron–glia interaction is known to play an important role in astroglial morphology, so the differences found here in astroglial shape of cells differentiated in CSF or P4-8F (Hatten, 1985; Emsley and Macklis, 2006) might be thereby explained. These results support our hypothesis of CSF promoting astrogliogenesis and probably are one possible explanation for the parallel increase of *Gfap* and *Nestin* mRNA during the first hours of differentiation in CSF. The coexpression of nestin and GFAP has recently been described in primary cultures of astroglial cells (Schmidt-Kastner and Humpel, 2002) and in astrocytes of organotypic slice cultures from rat cortex (Sergent-Tanguy et al., 2006). Thereby, nestin$^+$/GFAP$^+$ cells were described as immature astrocytes in which the expression of nestin did not necessarily predict an active state of proliferation (Schmidt-Kastner and Humpel, 2002). This observation offers a possible explanation for our finding that, with RT-PCR, no significant decrease of *Nestin* under the initial value could be determined after 72 hr of differentiation even when we found only very few Ki67$^+$ cells in CSF at that time point of differentiation. In P4-8F media, *Nestin* expression showed no transient increase but decreased significantly at 72 hr of differentiation. These finding might be due to the fact that, compared with CSF, a lower amount of cells differentiate into astrocytes. In addition, some signals required for glial maturation might be present only in P4-8F media, leading to a quicker switch in intermediate filament protein expression and to a shorter time of nestin/GFAP coexpression.

Several recent studies have suggested that the transplantation of NSCs via CSF could be a promising alternative to the direct transplantation of NSCs into the CNS (Wu et al., 2002a,b; Bai et al., 2003; Ohta et al., 2004). Thus, operation risks could be minimized, and a widespread distribution of NSCs into the possibly multifocally lesioned CNS could be achieved. At the same time, cell distribution could be restricted to the primarily affected organ, and side effects arising from peripherally applied cells could be avoided (Habisch et al., 2007; Lepore and Maragakis, 2007; Mazzini et al., 2008). Interestingly, injected NSCs tend to attach primarily to the lesion site, from which they invade the CNS tissue (Wu et al., 2002a,b; Bai et al., 2003; Ohta et al., 2004). Similar findings have been described for neural progenitors transplanted directly into the brain tissue, where they migrated toward localized (e.g., stroke) or diffuse (e.g., demyelinated) areas of brain damage (Fricker et al., 1999; Olstorn et al., 2007), most likely because of the expression of chemoattractants by the brain lesion or disease cell population (Belmadani et al., 2006). Contrary to these findings, Habisch et al. (2007) did not find relevant migration of transplanted human stem cells into the spinal cord in an ALS mouse model and, consistently, did not detect any motor improvement or effects on survival after intrathecal application of human mesoderm-derived NSCs. A low survival rate of injected cells because of the low nutrition content of CSF was hypothesized (Habisch et al., 2007), contradicting previous studies suggesting that CSF provides a beneficial environment for cell survival and proliferation after intraventricular transplantation (Wu et al., 2002a; Bai et al., 2003). In these studies, fetal NSCs were injected into the fourth ventricle of spinal cord-lesioned rats, and a good survival of grafted cells within the CSF was found (Wu et al., 2002a; Bai et al., 2003). In contrast to these results, it has previously been reported that pathologically modified CNS from patients with primary-progressive multiple sclerosis and Parkinson's disease leads to apoptosis in fetal rodent cortical neurons in primary cultures and to cell death and growth inhibition in PC12 cells (Alcazar et al., 1998; Mandybur et al., 2003). It is not known what influence this might have on NSCs. It remains therefore unclear whether NSCs would survive a nontraumatic transplantation via CSF in patients with neurodegenerative disorders such as Parkinson's disease or ALS. Indeed, markedly increased levels of proinflammatory prostaglandins such as PGE_2 and cytokines such as TNF-α, interferon-γ, and IL-1β were recently determined in the CSF of Parkinson's disease and ALS patients (Almer et al., 2002; Teismann and Schulz, 2004). Their influence on NSCs still has to be determined.

Recently, several research groups reported on the pivotal importance of CSF in brain development and in survival, proliferation, and differentiation of neuroectodermal stem cells (Mashayekhi et al., 2002; Gato et al., 2004, 2005; Martin et al., 2006; Bachy et al., 2008). All studies used embryonic CSF for these developmental studies, but, because of the above-discussed discrepancies between embryonic and adult CSF, comparisons with our data on adult CSF should be made cautiously. CSF circulation and pressure are known to play an important role in normal development of the CNS as well as the CSF itself, with its components (Gato and Desmond, 2009). In one study on chick embryos, embryonic avian CSF indeed promoted survival of NSCs in mesencephalic explants but induced neurogenesis and proliferation, with is contrary to our present findings, albeit in a totally different cell system (Gato et al., 2005). There are known differences in early brain development between birds, such as chickens, and mammals, such as rats or humans, with the mesencephalon growing fastest in birds and the forebrain growing fastest in mammals (Gato and Desmond, 2009). Because the early brain development is similar in rat and human (Gato and Desmond, 2009), we think that the data presented on rat NSCs have clinical relevance. Nevertheless, the results should be reproduced for human NSCs in further studies. Owing to the fact that embryonic CSF of human origin is hardly available for research purposes, a direct comparison of human embryonic and adult CSF with respect to their influences on NSC behavior is not possible, and whether embryonic or adult human CSFs have different effects on stem cell behavior remains unknown. An alternative use of rat embryonic CSF is in our eyes not practicable, because one can obtain only 5–15 μl CSF from one rat embryo (Miyan et al., 2006), which means, together with our need for about 50 ml for one set of experiments, that hundreds of individuals would have had to be sacrificed for sufficient amounts of CSF. This seemed not only impracticable but also ethically not justifiable. The use of human CSF of NPH patients seemed the only practicable source of large enough amounts of CSF with normal parameters in all measurable laboratory tests (see Materials and Methods). The decision to use CSF of NPH patients was also supported by the fact that hydrocephalic CSF of diseases with an elevated ventricular CSF pressure and disturbed CSF circulation because of, for example, cerebral aqueduct stenosis seems to alter the development of the CNS in animal models (Mashayekhi et al., 2002; Owen-Lynch et al., 2003). It is known that lumbar CSF is distinct from ventricular CSF because of passive diffusion processes across the blood–CSF barrier and suggested active secretion processes (Miyan et al., 2003) in the craniocaudal circulation. Thus, all CSF effects described here can be attributed only to leptomeningeal CSF. Resolving whether ventricular CSF has the same effects on NSC behavior is so far elusive. The use of CSF from ventricular drainage, however, is unfortunately problematic. First, ventricular drainages are brought into action in ill organisms with obstructed CSF circulation (for example, cerebral aqueduct stenosis) or other reasons for elevated brain pressure with defective blood–brain and blood–CSF barrier (for example, after major stroke or after intracerebral bleedings or inoperable brain tumors), so the goal of using healthy, normal CSF would be contradicted. Second, CSF from ventricular drainages often has blood contamination and is often altered by inflammatory processes and therefore cannot be used for the examination of effects of healthy CSF.

In summary, our results demonstrate that adult human leptomeningeal CSF has a trophic influence on fetal NSCs. Survival, neurite outgrowth, and differentiation primarily to astroglia were promoted by CSF, whereas neurogenesis and oligodengrogenesis were inhibited. An attachment of injected NSCs to the ventricle wall, where they were injected, has been reported from previous studies (Wu et al., 2002a; Habisch et al., 2007). The rapid differentiation of NSCs and the accelerated loss of stem cell potential that we found may impede sufficient migration into the CNS. Which factors in CSF lead to the observed differences in NSC behavior in comparison with differentiation in standard culture media is so far unclear, but differences in albumin content can be excluded, insofar as the used P4-8F medium has an albumin content matching physiological conditions of healthy adult CSF (see Materials and Methods).

One potential factor mediating the CSF effects seen is bone morphogenic proteins (BMPs), some of which are known to be present at least in bovine CSF (Dattatreyamurty et al., 2001; Moon et al., 2009). Cotreatment of our cultures with the BMP antagonist noggin reversed some of the CSF effects completely (mainly cell survival during expansion and differentiation, neurite branching) but did not influence CSF action on self-renewing potential as measured by BrdU staining. We therefore conclude that BMPs may well be part of the factors in CSF influencing NSC behavior at least in our in vitro system, but other as yet unknown factors have to play an additional role. Future experiments determining which contents in adult CSF influence the behavior of NSCs and investigating possibilities to influence the differentiation behavior of NSCs in CSF are needed. In addition, further studies on the influence of CSF from the diseased CNS (for example, from stroke patients, Parkinson's disease patients) on NSCs are warranted to make their transplantation via CSF a real therapeutic option for patients with neurodegenerative disorders.

ACKNOWLEDGMENTS

The authors thank the Departments of Surgery and Clinical Chemistry of the EMAU for allowing us to use parts of their equipment. We thank Sigrid Peters for expert technical assistance.

REFERENCES

Alcazar A, Regidor I, Masjuan J, Salinas M, Alvarez-Cermeno JC. 1998. Induction of apoptosis by cerebrospinal fluid from patients with primary-progressive multiple sclerosis in cultured neurons. Neurosci Lett 255:75–78.

Almer G, Teismann P, Stevic Z, Halaschek-Wiener J, Deecke L, Kostic V, Przedborski S. 2002. Increased levels of the pro-inflammatory prostaglandin PGE2 in CSF from ALS patients. Neurology 58:1277–1279.

Alvarez-Buylla A, Garcia-Verdugo JM. 2002. Neurogenesis in adult subventricular zone. J Neurosci 22:629–634.

Bachy I, Kozyraki R, Wassef M. 2008. The particles of the embryonic cerebrospinal fluid: how could they influence brain development? Brain Res Bull 75:289–294.

Bai H, Suzuki Y, Noda T, Wu S, Kataoka K, Kitada M, Ohta M, Chou H, Ide C. 2003. Dissemination and proliferation of neural stem cells on the spinal cord by injection into the fourth ventricle of the rat: a method for cell transplantation. J Neurosci Methods 124:181–187.

Bain G, Kitchens D, Yao M, Huettner JE, Gottlieb DI. 1995. Embryonic stem cells express neuronal properties in vitro. Dev Biol 168:342–357.

Belmadani A, Tran PB, Ren D, Miller RJ. 2006. Chemokines regulate the migration of neural progenitors to sites of neuroinflammation. J Neurosci 26:3182–3191.

Cai J, Limke TL, Ginis I, Rao MS. 2003. Identifying and tracking neural stem cells. Blood Cells Mol Dis 31:18–27.

Chu K, Kim M, Park KI, Jeong SW, Park HK, Jung KH, Lee ST, Kang L, Lee K, Park DK, Kim SU, Roh JK. 2004. Human neural stem cells improve sensorimotor deficits in the adult rat brain with experimental focal ischemia. Brain Res 1016:145–153.

Corti S, Locatelli F, Papadimitriou D, Del Bo R, Nizzardo M, Nardini M, Donadoni C, Salani S, Fortunato F, Strazzer S, Bresolin N, Comi GP. 2007. Neural stem cells LewisX$^+$ CXCR4$^+$ modify disease progression in an amyotrophic lateral sclerosis model. Brain 130:1289–1305.

Darsalia V, Kallur T, Kokaia Z. 2007. Survival, migration and neuronal differentiation of human fetal striatal and cortical neural stem cells grafted in stroke-damaged rat striatum. Eur J Neurosci 26:605–614.

Dattatreyamurty B, Roux E, Horbinski C, Kaplan PL, Robak LA, Beck HN, Lein P, Higgins D, Chandrasekaran V. 2001. Cerebrospinal fluid contains biologically active bone morphogenetic protein-7. Exp Neurol 172:273–281.

Eisch AJ, Mandyam CD. 2007. Adult neurogenesis: can analysis of cell cycle proteins move us "beyond BrdU"? Curr Pharm Biotechnol 8:147–165.

Emsley JG, Macklis JD. 2006. Astroglial heterogeneity closely reflects the neuronal-defined anatomy of the adult murine CNS. Neuron Glia Biol 2:175–186.

Fricker RA, Carpenter MK, Winkler C, Greco C, Gates MA, Bjorklund A. 1999. Site-specific migration and neuronal differentiation of human neural progenitor cells after transplantation in the adult rat brain. J Neurosci 19:5990–6005.

Gage FH. 2000. Mammalian neural stem cells. Science 287:1433–1438.

Gato A, Desmond ME. 2009. Why the embryo still matters: CSF and the neuroepithelium as interdependent regulators of embryonic brain growth, morphogenesis and histiogenesis. Dev Biol 327:263–272.

Gato A, Martin P, Alonso MI, Martin C, Pulgar MA, Moro JA. 2004. Analysis of cerebrospinal fluid protein composition in early developmental stages in chick embryos. J Exp Zool 301:280–289.

Gato A, Moro JA, Alonso MI, Bueno D, De La Mano A, Martin C. 2005. Embryonic cerebrospinal fluid regulates neuroepithelial survival, proliferation, and neurogenesis in chick embryos. Anat Rec 284:475–484.

Gerdes J, Schwab U, Lemke H, Stein H. 1983. Production of a mouse monoclonal antibody reactive with a human nuclear antigen associated with cell proliferation. Int J Cancer 31:13–20.

Gerdes J, Lemke H, Baisch H, Wacker HH, Schwab U, Stein H. 1984. Cell cycle analysis of a cell proliferation-associated human nuclear antigen defined by the monoclonal antibody Ki-67. J Immunol 133:1710–1715.

Habisch HJ, Janowski M, Binder D, Kuzma-Kozakiewicz M, Widmann A, Habich A, Schwalenstocker B, Hermann A, Brenner R, Lukomska B, Domanska-Janik K, Ludolph AC, Storch A. 2007. Intrathecal application of neuroectodermally converted stem cells into a mouse model of ALS: limited intraparenchymal migration and survival narrows therapeutic effects. J Neural Transmiss (in press).

Hatten ME. 1985. Neuronal regulation of astroglial morphology and proliferation in vitro. J Cell Biol 100:384–396.

Hermann A, Gastl R, Liebau S, Popa MO, Fiedler J, Boehm BO, Maisel M, Lerche H, Schwarz J, Brenner R, Storch A. 2004. Efficient generation of neural stem cell-like cells from adult human bone marrow stromal cells. J Cell Sci 117:4411–4422.

Jain M, Armstrong RJ, Elneil S, Barker RA. 2006. Transplanted human neural precursor cells migrate widely but show no lesion-specific tropism in the 6-hydroxydopamine rat model of Parkinson's disease. Cell Transplant 15:579–593.

Jeong SW, Chu K, Jung KH, Kim SU, Kim M, Roh JK. 2003. Human neural stem cell transplantation promotes functional recovery in rats with experimental intracerebral hemorrhage. Stroke J Cereb Circ 34:2258–2263.

Johanson CE, Duncan JA 3rd, Klinge PM, Brinker T, Stopa EG, Silverberg GD. 2008. Multiplicity of cerebrospinal fluid functions: new challenges in health and disease. Cerebrospinal Fluid Res 5:10.

Johansson CB, Momma S, Clarke DL, Risling M, Lendahl U, Frisen J. 1999. Identification of a neural stem cell in the adult mammalian central nervous system. Cell 96:25–34.

Kawasaki H, Mizuseki K, Nishikawa S, Kaneko S, Kuwana Y, Nakanishi S, Nishikawa SI, Sasai Y. 2000. Induction of midbrain dopaminergic neurons from ES cells by stromal cell-derived inducing activity. Neuron 28:31–40.

Kawasaki H, Suemori H, Mizuseki K, Watanabe K, Urano F, Ichinose H, Haruta M, Takahashi M, Yoshikawa K, Nishikawa S, Nakatsuji N, Sasai Y. 2002. Generation of dopaminergic neurons and pigmented epithelia from primate ES cells by stromal cell-derived inducing activity. Proc Natl Acad Sci U S A 99:1580–1585.

Kitayama T, Onitsuka Y, Song L, Morioka N, Morita K, Dohi T. 2007. Assessing an eating disorder induced by 6-OHDA and the possibility of nerve regeneration therapy by transplantation of neural progenitor cells in rats. Nihon Shinkei Seishin Yakurigaku Zasshi 27:109–116.

Lee HJ, Kim KS, Kim EJ, Choi HB, Lee KH, Park IH, Ko Y, Jeong SW, Kim SU. 2007. Brain transplantation of immortalized human neural stem cells promotes functional recovery in mouse intracerebral hemorrhage stroke model. Stem Cells 25:1204–1212.

Lee SH, Lumelsky N, Studer L, Auerbach JM, McKay RD. 2000. Efficient generation of midbrain and hindbrain neurons from mouse embryonic stem cells. Nat Biotechnol 18:675–679.

Leite MC, Galland F, Brolese G, Guerra MC, Bortolotto JW, Freitas R, Almeida LM, Gottfried C, Goncalves CA. 2008. A simple, sensitive and widely applicable ELISA for S100B: methodological features of the measurement of this glial protein. J Neurosci Methods 169:93–99.

Lepore AC, Maragakis NJ. 2007. Targeted stem cell transplantation strategies in ALS. Neurochem Int 50:966–975.

Lepore AC, Neuhuber B, Connors TM, Han SS, Liu Y, Daniels MP, Rao MS, Fischer I. 2006. Long-term fate of neural precursor cells following transplantation into developing and adult CNS. Neuroscience 142:287–304.

Livak KJ, Schmittgen TD. 2001. Analysis of relative gene expression data using real-time quantitative PCR and the 2(–Delta Delta C_T) method. Methods 25:402–408.

Magavi SS, Leavitt BR, Macklis JD. 2000. Induction of neurogenesis in the neocortex of adult mice. Nature 405:951–955.

Mandybur GT, Miyagi Y, Yin W, Perkins E, Zhang JH. 2003. Cytotoxicity of ventricular cerebrospinal fluid from Parkinson patients: correlation with clinical profiles and neurochemistry. Neurol Res 25:104–111.

Martin C, Bueno D, Alonso MI, Moro JA, Callejo S, Parada C, Martin P, Carnicero E, Gato A. 2006. FGF2 plays a key role in embryonic cerebrospinal fluid trophic properties over chick embryo neuroepithelial stem cells. Dev Biol 297:402–416.

Martin LJ, Liu Z. 2007. Adult olfactory bulb neural precursor cell grafts provide temporary protection from motor neuron degeneration, improve motor function, and extend survival in amyotrophic lateral sclerosis mice. J Neuropathol Exp Neurol 66:1002–1018.

Mashayekhi F, Draper CE, Bannister CM, Pourghasem M, Owen-Lynch PJ, Miyan JA. 2002. Deficient cortical development in the hydrocephalic Texas (H-Tx) rat: a role for CSF. Brain 125:1859–1874.

Mazzini L, Mareschi K, Ferrero I, Vassallo E, Oliveri G, Nasuelli N, Oggioni GD, Testa L, Fagioli F. 2008. Stem cell treatment in amyotrophic lateral sclerosis. J Neurol Sci 265:78–83.

McKay R. 1997. Stem cells in the central nervous system. Science 276:66–71.

Milosevic J, Storch A, Schwarz J. 2004. Spontaneous apoptosis in murine free-floating neurospheres. Exp Cell Res 294:9–17.

Miyan JA, Nabiyouni M, Zendah M. 2003. Development of the brain: a vital role for cerebrospinal fluid. Can J Physiol Pharmacol 81:317–328.

Miyan JA, Zendah M, Mashayekhi F, Owen-Lynch PJ. 2006. Cerebrospinal fluid supports viability and proliferation of cortical cells in vitro, mirroring in vivo development. Cerebrospinal Fluid Res 3:2.

Moon BS, Yoon JY, Kim MY, Lee SH, Choi T, Choi KY. 2009. Bone morphogenetic protein 4 stimulates neuronal differentiation of neuronal stem cells through the ERK pathway. Exp Mol Med 41:116–125.

Nordin C, Gupta RC, Sjodin I. 2007. Cerebrospinal fluid amino acids in pathological gamblers and healthy controls. Neuropsychobiology 56:152–158.

Ohta M, Suzuki Y, Noda T, Kataoka K, Chou H, Ishikawa N, Kitada M, Matsumoto N, Dezawa M, Suzuki S, Ide C. 2004. Implantation of neural stem cells via cerebrospinal fluid into the injured root. Neuroreport 15:1249–1253.

Olstorn H, Moe MC, Roste GK, Bueters T, Langmoen IA. 2007. Transplantation of stem cells from the adult human brain to the adult rat brain. Neurosurgery 60:1089–1098; discussion 1098–1089.

Owen-Lynch PJ, Draper CE, Mashayekhi F, Bannister CM, Miyan JA. 2003. Defective cell cycle control underlies abnormal cortical development in the hydrocephalic Texas rat. Brain 126:623–631.

Parada C, Gato A, Bueno D. 2005. Mammalian embryonic cerebrospinal fluid proteome has greater apolipoprotein and enzyme pattern complexity than the avian proteome. J Proteome Res 4:2420–2428.

Reynolds BA, Weiss S. 1992. Generation of neurons and astrocytes from isolated cells of the adult mammalian central nervous system. Science 255:1707–1710.

Rietze RL, Valcanis H, Brooker GF, Thomas T, Voss AK, Bartlett PF. 2001. Purification of a pluripotent neural stem cell from the adult mouse brain. Nature 412:736–739.

Sabolek M, Herborg A, Schwarz J, Storch A. 2006. Dexamethasone blocks astroglial differentiation from neural precursor cells. Neuroreport 17:1719–1723.

Schmidt-Kastner R, Humpel C. 2002. Nestin expression persists in astrocytes of organotypic slice cultures from rat cortex. Int J Dev Neurosci 20:29–38.

Sergent-Tanguy S, Michel DC, Neveu I, Naveilhan P. 2006. Long-lasting coexpression of nestin and glial fibrillary acidic protein in primary cultures of astroglial cells with a major participation of nestin$^+$/GFAP$^-$ cells in cell proliferation. J Neurosci Res 83:1515–1524.

Shihabuddin LS, Horner PJ, Ray J, Gage FH. 2000. Adult spinal cord stem cells generate neurons after transplantation in the adult dentate gyrus. J Neurosci 20:8727–8735.

Sievertzon M, Wirta V, Mercer A, Meletis K, Erlandsson R, Wikstrom L, Frisen J, Lundeberg J. 2005. Transcriptome analysis in primary neural stem cells using a tag cDNA amplification method. BMC Neurosci 6:28.

Storch A, Paul G, Csete M, Boehm BO, Carvey PM, Kupsch A, Schwarz J. 2001. Long-term proliferation and dopaminergic differentiation of human mesencephalic neural precursor cells. Exp Neurol 170:317–325.

Storch A, Lester HA, Boehm BO, Schwarz J. 2003. Functional characterization of dopaminergic neurons derived from rodent mesencephalic progenitor cells. J Chem Neuroanat 26:133–142.

Storch A, Sabolek M, Milosevic J, Schwarz SC, Schwarz J. 2004. Midbrain-derived neural stem cells: from basic science to therapeutic approaches. Cell Tissue Res 318:15–22.

Svendsen CN, Caldwell MA, Shen J, ter Borg MG, Rosser AE, Tyers P, Karmiol S, Dunnett SB. 1997. Long-term survival of human central nervous system progenitor cells transplanted into a rat model of Parkinson's disease. Exp Neurol 148:135–146.

Svendsen CN, Caldwell MA, Ostenfeld T. 1999. Human neural stem cells: isolation, expansion and transplantation. Brain Pathol 9:499–513.

Teismann P, Schulz JB. 2004. Cellular pathology of Parkinson's disease: astrocytes, microglia, and inflammation. Cell Tissue Res 318:149–161.

Tramontin AD, Garcia-Verdugo JM, Lim DA, Alvarez-Buylla A. 2003. Postnatal development of radial glia and the ventricular zone (VZ): a continuum of the neural stem cell compartment. Cereb Cortex 13:580–587.

Vazey EM, Chen K, Hughes SM, Connor B. 2006. Transplanted adult neural progenitor cells survive, differentiate and reduce motor function impairment in a rodent model of Huntington's disease. Exp Neurol 199:384–396.

Wei P, Liu J, Zhou HL, Han ZT, Wu QY, Pang JX, Liu S, Wang TH. 2007. Effects of engrafted neural stem cells derived from GFP transgenic mice in Parkinson's diseases rats. Neurosci Lett 419:49–54.

Wu S, Suzuki Y, Kitada M, Kataoka K, Kitaura M, Chou H, Nishimura Y, Ide C. 2002a. New method for transplantation of neurosphere cells into injured spinal cord through cerebrospinal fluid in rat. Neurosci Lett 318:81–84.

Wu S, Suzuki Y, Noda T, Bai H, Kitada M, Kataoka K, Nishimura Y, Ide C. 2002b. Immunohistochemical and electron microscopic study of invasion and differentiation in spinal cord lesion of neural stem cells grafted through cerebrospinal fluid in rat. J Neurosci Res 69:940–945.

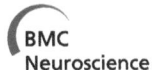

RESEARCH ARTICLE

Open Access

Cerebrospinal fluid promotes survival and astroglial differentiation of adult human neural progenitor cells but inhibits proliferation and neuronal differentiation

Judith Buddensiek[1], Alexander Dressel[1], Michael Kowalski[1], Uwe Runge[1], Henry Schroeder[2], Andreas Hermann[3], Matthias Kirsch[4], Alexander Storch[3], Michael Sabolek[1*]

Abstract

Background: Neural stem cells (NSCs) are a promising source for cell replacement therapies for neurological diseases. Growing evidence suggests an important role of cerebrospinal fluid (CSF) not only on neuroectodermal cells during brain development but also on the survival, proliferation and fate specification of NSCs in the adult brain. Existing in vitro studies focused on embryonic cell lines and embryonic CSF. We therefore studied the effects of adult human leptomeningeal CSF on the behaviour of adult human NSCs (ahNSCs).

Results: Adult CSF increased the survival rate of adult human NSCs compared to standard serum free culture media during both stem cell maintenance and differentiation. The presence of CSF promoted differentiation of NSCs leading to a faster loss of their self-renewal capacity as it is measured by the proliferation markers Ki67 and BrdU and stronger cell extension outgrowth with longer and more cell extensions per cell. After differentiation in CSF, we found a larger number of GFAP$^+$ astroglial cells compared to differentiation in standard culture media and a lower number of β-tubulin III$^+$ neuronal cells.

Conclusions: Our data demonstrate that adult human leptomeningeal CSF creates a beneficial environment for the survival and differentiation of adult human NSCs. Adult CSF is *in vitro* a strong glial differentiation stimulus and leads to a rapid loss of stem cell potential.

Background

Neural stem cells (NSCs) are a promising source for cell replacement therapies in the brain and the spinal cord [1]. It is common knowledge that NSCs can be extracted from fetal brain [2-4] or generated from embryonic stem cells [2,5-8]. Furthermore, NSCs can also be isolated from different regions of the adult brain such as the hippocampus and the subventricular zone and from some non-neurogenic regions such as the spinal cord [2,3,9-13] or the periventricular regions of the whole neuroaxis [14]. NSCs are able to replicate and generate all neuroectodermal lineages, namely neurons, astroglia and oligodendroglia [2,3,15]. During *in vitro* expansion,

NSCs grow in so-called "neurospheres" or adherent cultures. Neurospheres are either multicellular aggregates or clones originating from one single cell depending on the cell density [3,9,11,15]. In previous studies, the isolation and successful long-term expansion of human NSCs from the adult hippocampus, the adult olfactory bulb and adult post-mortem tissues have been reported [16-20]. In these studies, ahNSCs have successfully been expanded for more than 30 population doublings using serum-free culture medium which is normally supplemented with the mitogenes epidermal growth factor (EGF) and fibroblast growth factor 2 (FGF-2). Removal of the mitogenes leads to spontaneous differentiation of adult NSCs into neurons, astroglia and oligondendroglia [16-20].

Investigations examining the influence of CSF and its contents on survival, proliferation and differentiation of

* Correspondence: michael.sabolek@uni-greifswald.de
[1]Department of Neurology, Ernst Moritz Arndt University of Greifswald, 17475 Greifswald, Germany

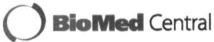

© 2010 Buddensiek et al; licensee BioMed Central Ltd. This is an Open Access article distributed under the terms of the Creative Commons Attribution License (http://creativecommons.org/licenses/by/2.0), which permits unrestricted use, distribution, and reproduction in any medium, provided the original work is properly cited.

NSCs were so far mostly performed with embryonic avian CSF [21-23]. In these investigations, NSCs cultured in CSF showed an increased survival rate and a higher number of BrdU positive, DNA synthesizing nuclei, compared to standard culture media. In addition a larger number of beta-tubulin III$^+$, immature neurons, has been detected compared to standard culture media, indicating a positive influence of embryonic avian CSF on neurogenesis. As there are well known differences between avian and mammalian CSF [24] with a much greater complexity of mammalian CSF, the transferability of these results to human conditions is not yet clear. Also, they might be a difference in between effects of adult CSF on NSCs and embryonic CSF effects. Still, this is not yet investigated, even though it has been suggested that CSF plays an important role not only during brain differentation but also for the survival, proliferation and differentiation of neuroectodermal stem cells in vivo [21-23,25-27]. In this present study we therefore used an in vitro cell system of adult human NSCs in culture as a model to investigate the effects of adult human CSF on NSC behaviour.

Results
CSF increases the survival rate of adult human NSCs
After in vitro expansion for at least three passages in standard media, NSCs were transferred to uncoated chamber slides and expanded in standard expansion medium or CSF for additional 72 h. Thereafter, cells were stained with Hoechst 33342 and propidiumiodid to determine the amount of necrotic cells. Our results showed a significantly higher survival rate of NSCs in CSF compared to standard expansion medium (see Materials and Methods) with 6.9 ± 1.9% of necrotic cells in CSF versus 46.0 ± 12.9% in expansion medium (P = 0.013; Fig. 1). Addition of the bone morphogenic protein (BMP) inhibitor Noggin did not significantly increase cell death rates compared to CSF without Noggin (5.2 ± 2.4% of necrotic cells, P = 0.54; Fig. 1). Similar results were obtained during in vitro differentiation with significantly higher survival rates in CSF compared to standard differentiation media: After 24 h in P4-8F media, 20.3 ± 2.6% of NSCs were found necrotic versus 10.1 ± 2.9% in CSF (P = 0.021). After 72 h, the proportion was 22.7 ± 7.5% versus 6.5 ± 0.8% for standard media versus CSF, respectively (P = 0.038; Fig. 2). Again, addition of Noggin to CSF had no significant influence on the cell death rate during differentiation for the first 24 h (2.4 ± 1.5% of necrotic cells, P = 0.09 when compared CSF with CSF plus Noggin condition; Fig. 2).

CSF inhibits proliferation of adult human NSCs
To determine the influence of adult human leptomeningeal CSF on self-renewal potential of adult NSCs, we used the proliferation markers Ki67 and BrdU as readouts. For this, after in vitro expansion of at least three passages, cells were transferred to uncoated chamber slides and expanded in culture medium or CSF. The self renewing potential was determined at 24 h (Ki67) and 72 h (BrdU) after media was changed. At each time point, the percentage of Ki67$^+$ and BrdU$^+$ NSCs was significantly higher in expansion medium compared to the one in CSF, representing a larger number of proliferating cells in expansion media. Hence, after 24 h Ki67 was detected in 20.4 ± 7.3% of NSCs expanded in standard medium compared to only 0.2 ± 0.01% of NSCs expanded in CSF (P = < 0.001; Fig. 3). For BrdU, we detected 42.8 ± 15.7 BrdU$^+$ cells/cm^2 in KO-DMEM, but only 2.4 ± 2.8 BrdU$^+$ cells/cm^2 in CSF (P = 0.023, Fig. 3).

CSF increases extension outgrowth velocity from adult human NSCs
We used the time course of extension outgrowth as a first measure of the differentiation process of NSCs in culture. Thus, following expansion for at least three passages in vitro NSCs were allowed to differentiate. Cells were plated onto PLL-coated chamber slides in either differentiation media or CSF. For investigating extension outgrowth, number and length of extensions were determined at 0, 3, 6, 24 and 72 h after starting the differentiation process. Comparing results in P4-8F and CSF, we found significantly longer and a significantly more cell extensions per cell in CSF. After 24 and 72 h the difference was significant as NSC neurites getting twice as long in CSF (mean length: 14.5 ± 2.6 and 33.2 ± 1.4 μm after 24 and 72 h, respectively) as in P4-8F (mean length: 7.7 ± 0.9 and 10.6 ± 3.2; P = 0.024 [24 h] and 0.001 [72 h]; Fig. 4). Significant more cell extensions were determined in CSF for the time points 6 h, 24 h and 72 h with an average number of 1.3 ± 0.0 cell extensions in CSF after 6 h compared to 1.2 ± 0.1 neuritis in P4-8F. After 24 h, the mean number of cell extensions was 1.5 ± 0.1 in CSF versus 1.2 ± 0.1 in P48F and after 72 hours cells had at an average of 2.0 ± 0.1 cell extensions in CSF compared to 1.5 ± 0.1 in P4-8F respectively.(P = 0.001, 0.008 and 0.005, respectively; Fig. 4).

CSF facilitates astrogliogenesis but inhibits neurogenesis from adult human NSCs
To investigate the question whether the presence of adult human leptomeningeal CSF does have an influence on astrogliogenesis, oligodendrogenesis or neurogenesis, adult NSCs were allowed to differentiate for 7 days on PLL-coated chamber slides in either standard differentiation media or CSF. After differentiation in standard media, 24.7 ± 1.7% of the cells were GFAP$^+$, in contrast

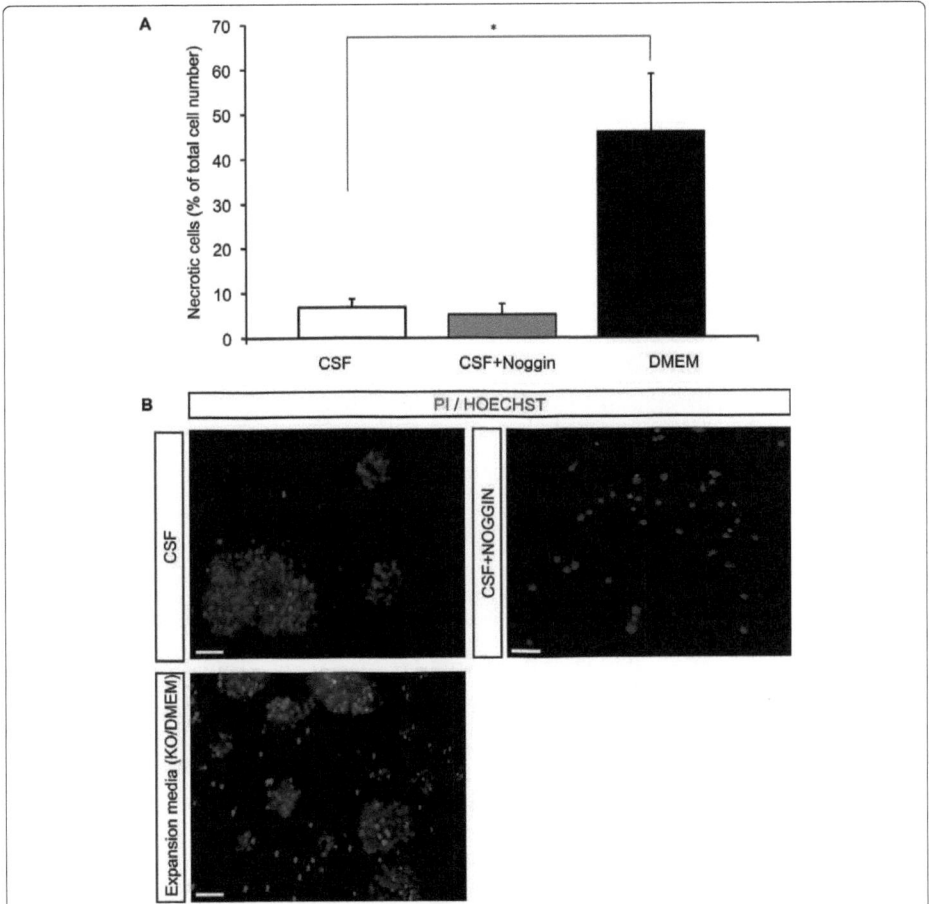

Figure 1 Survival rate of human adult NSCs during expansion. **A**, The percentage of necrotic NSCs expanded in culture medium supplemented with EGF and FGF-2 in comparison to CSF with or without 150 ng/ml Noggin was determined 72 hours after starting the expansion process. Values represent the mean ± S.E.M from at least three independent experiments. * indicates $P < 0.05$ and ** $P < 0.01$ compared to each corresponding value in CSF. **B**, Representative microphotographs demonstrating the influence of CSF on survival rate of NSCs. For immunostainings, dead cells were stained with propidiumiodid. Nuclei were counterstained with Hoechst 33342. The upper panel shows NSCs expanded in CSF (left photograph) and CSF+Noggin (right photograph), the lower panel shows NSCs expanded in expansion media supplemented with EGF and FGF. Scale bar = 50 μm.

to 37.8 ± 7.8 GFAP$^+$ cells in CSF ($P = 0.014$; Fig. 5). The values for GalC$^+$ oligodendroglial cells and MAP2$^+$ neurons were 8.2 ± 2.6% GalC$^+$ and 0.2 ± 1.7 MAP2$^+$ cells in standard media and 7.0 ± 1.5 GalC$^+$ and 0.4 ± 0.6 MAP2$^+$ cells in CSF ($P > 0.05$). The low percentage of MAP2$^+$ cells in standard media and CSF is most likely caused by the lack of fully differentiated phenotypes, as MAP2 represents a marker for mature neurons. Staining against the neuronal marker protein β-tubulin III, a marker for immature neurons, revealed 8.7 ± 3.6% β-tubulin III$^+$ cells in CSF compared to 30.7 ± 8.4 β-tubulin III$^+$ cells in standard media ($P = 0.014$).

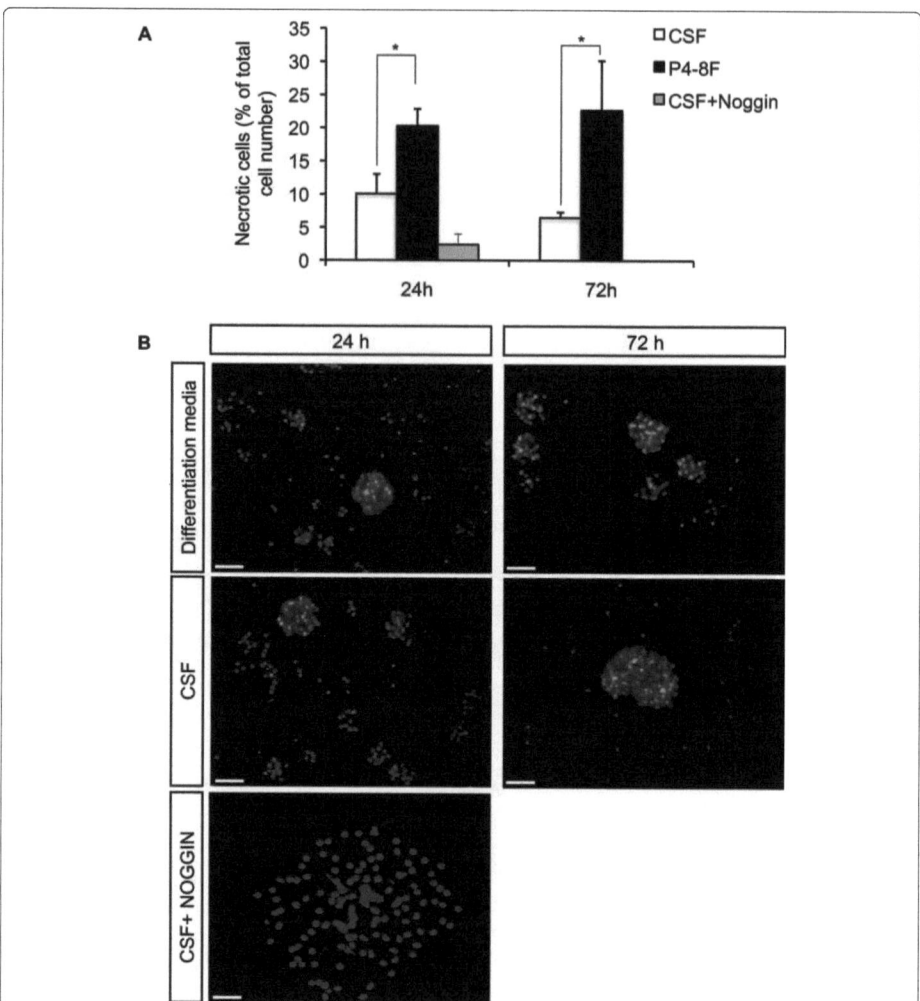

Figure 2 Survival rate of adult human NSCs during proliferation. **A**, The percentage of necrotic NSCs was determined at 24 and 72 hours after differentiation on PLL-coated chamber slides in P4-8F or CSF with or without 150 ng/ml Noggin. Values represent the mean ± S.E.M from at least three independent experiments. * indicates $P < 0.05$ and ** $P < 0.01$ compared to each corresponding value in CSF. **B**, Representative microphotographs demonstrating the influence of CSF on the survival rate of NSCs. For immunostainings, dead cells were stained with propidiumiodid. Nuclei were counterstained with Hoechst 33342. The upper panel shows NSCs differentiated in differentiation media P4-8F, the middle panel shows NSCs differentiated in CSF, and the lower panel shows NSCs differentiated in CSF+Noggin. Scale bar = 50 μm.

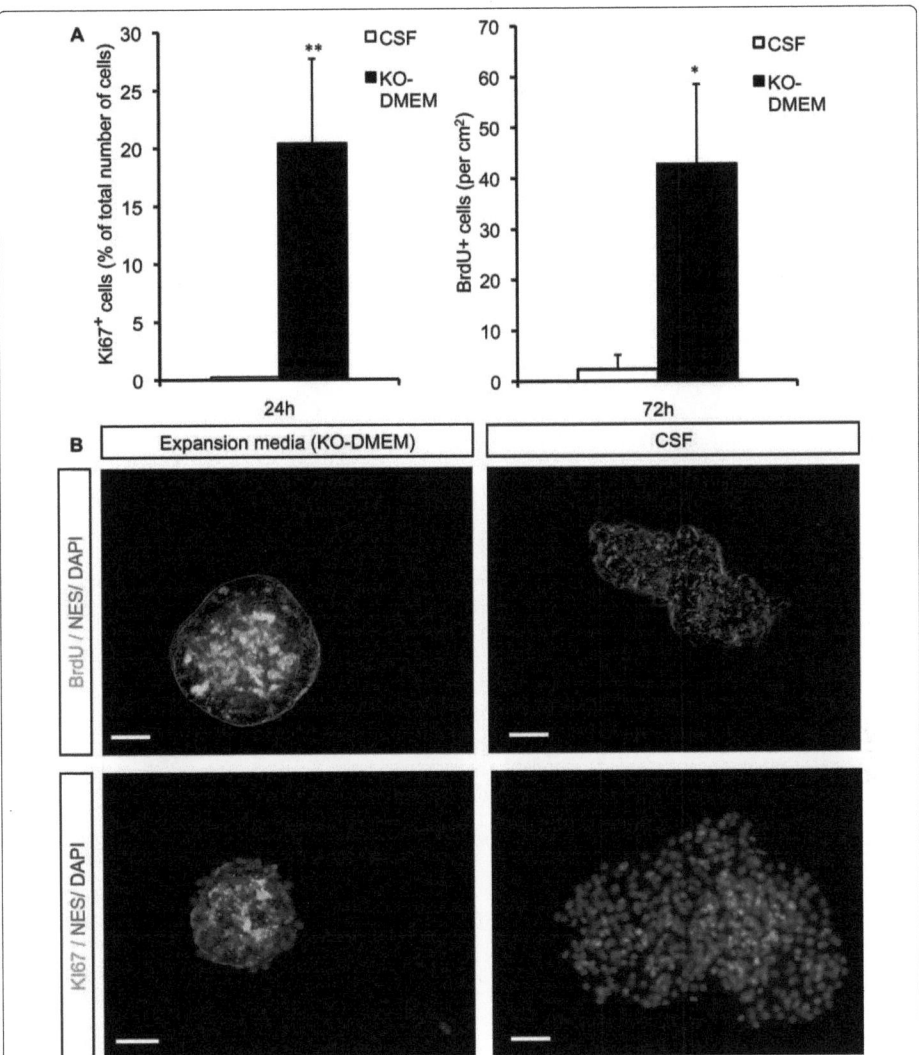

Figure 3 Investigation of cell proliferation in adult human NSCs during expansion. The portion of NSCs with potential to self renewal expanded in culture medium supplemented with EGF and FGF-2 or CSF without additional growth factors was determined 24 and 72 hours after medium change. **A**, Percentage of Ki67$^+$ cells after 24 h, number of BrdU$^+$ cells per cm^2 after 72 h. Values represent the mean ± S.E.M from at least three independent experiments. *indicates $P < 0.05$ and ** $P < 0.01$ compared to each corresponding value in CSF. **B**, Representative microphotographs demonstrating the influence of CSF on proliferation markers in NSCs. For immunostainings cells were stained with anti-BrdU (upper panel) and anti-Ki67 (lower panel) and anti-Nestin (upper and lower panel). Nuclei were counterstained with DAPI (lower panel). Altered morphology of neurospheres with CSF treatment (right panel) is most likely due to the beginning differentiation process. Scale bar = 50 μm.

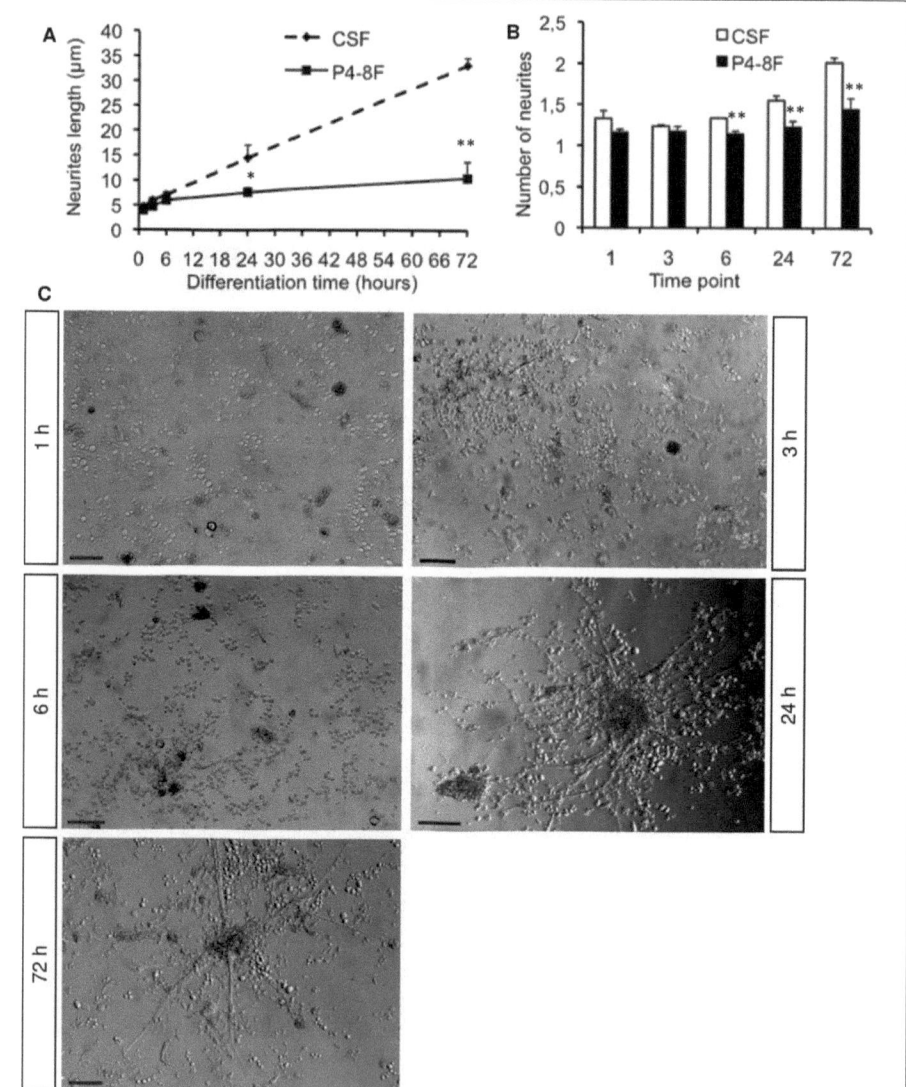

Figure 4 Cell extension outgrowth in adult human NSCs. **A**, Length of cell extensions (μm) after 1, 3, 6, 24, 72 hours of differentiation in P4-8F or adult human CSF. **B**, Number of cell extensions at 1, 3, 6, 24, 72 hours of differentiation in P4-8F or human adult CSF. **A and B**, Values represent the mean ± S.E.M from at least three independent experiments. * indicates $P < 0.05$ compared to each corresponding value in CSF. **C**, Representative microphotographs showing cell morphology after 1, 3, 6, 24, 72 hours of differentiation in CSF. Scale bar = 50 μm.

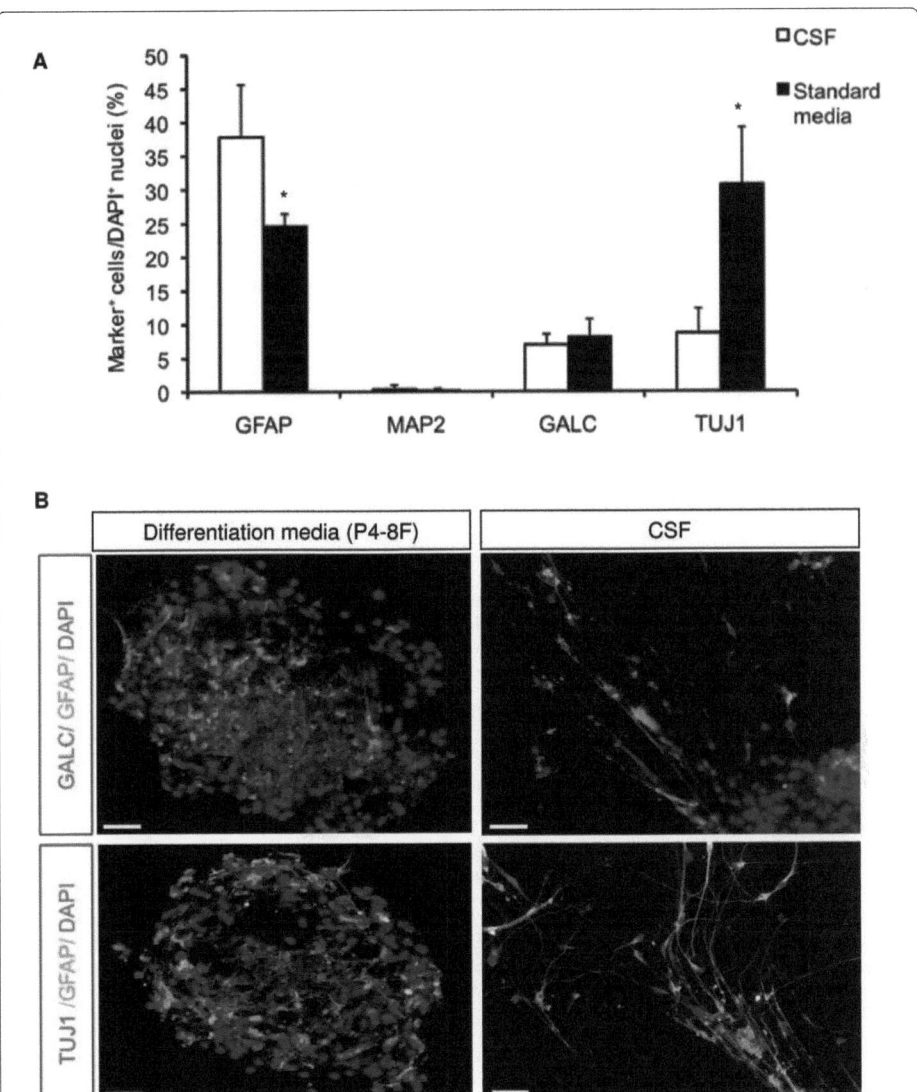

Figure 5 Neurogenesis and gliogenesis from adult human NSCs. A, The percentage of GFAP+, MAP2ab+, β-tubulin III and GALC+ cells after differentiation for 10 to 14 days in KO/DMEM or CSF. Results are mean values ± S.E.M from at least three independent experiments. * indicates $P < 0.05$ compared to each corresponding value in CSF. **B**, Representative microphotographs demonstrating the effects of CSF on neuronal and glial differentiation of ahNSCs 10 to 14 days after initiation of the differentiation process. Cells were stained with anti-GFAP, anti-β-tubulin III and anti-GALC. Nuclei were counterstained with DAPI. Scale bar = 50 μm.

Discussion

There is growing evidence that CSF plays an important role in physiological as well as pathophysiological processes of the brain including adult neurogenesis [28-30]. In a very recent study of our group, we found adult human leptomeningeal CSF being a promotor of survival, differentiation and astrogliogenesis of fetal NSCs from rat [31]. The influence of CSF on adult NSCs remains however still enigmatic. In this study we therefore used human adult NSCs as an *in vitro* model to study the effects of adult leptomeningeal CSF on NSC behaviour including survival, self renewal and differentiation. The central finding of our study is that *in vitro*, adult CSF promotes survival and differentiation of ahNSCs, but drives the differentiation process towards astrogliogenesis. In accordance with these findings, the loss of stem cell potential is accelerated when cultured in adult CSF. These findings suggest that adult CSF contains key factors involved in the control of cellular proliferation and differentiation processes. This assumption is supported by *in vivo* findings, demonstrating that adult NSCs of the subventricular zone have transitory contact with the ventricular brain cavity and many of them still posses one microcilia which extends into the CSF [32-35]. In addition, it is known from previous studies [21-23] that embryonic CSF has a trophic influence on survival and differentiation of NSCs. However, the loss of stem cell potential is decelerated, which is contradictory to our findings in adult CSF and may explain the abundance of post-mitotic cells in adult CNS.

Based on the knowledge of embryonic CSF studies, it has already been postulated that diffusible factors in embryonic CSF regulate the three basic cellular behavioural parameters of neuroephitelial stem cells and that embryonic CSF may play a key role in brain development *in vivo* [23].

However, how CSF influences neuroectodermal cells during development remains enigmatic, but the components contained in CSF as well as CSF pressure and flow seem to play an important role [26,36]. Regarding the components of CSF influencing neuroectodermal cell behaviour, recent investigations concentrated mainly on proteins, "membranous particles" and amino acids but also on growth factors such as FGF2 [21,24,25,36,37]. In avian and human CSF, many proteins with a known influence on cell survival, neural and glial differentiation, proliferation and signal transduction were found (such as transthyretin, serin, retinol binding protein, heparan sulfate, several apolipoproteins, and FGF2) [22,24,25]. Although it has also been demonstrated that the protein composition of embryonic CSF is more complex than that of adult CSF [22], our results indicate that adult CSF has the capacity to influence the behaviour of adult NSCs in the adult brain, too.

CSF as a beneficial environment for cell survival and growth has also been postulated by *in vivo* studies, investigating for example the behaviour of fetal NSCs after injection in the fourth ventricle of spinal cord lesioned rats with a good survival of grafted cells within the CSF [38,39], as well as in a recent *in vitro* study of our own group with fetal rat NSCs [31]. In the present study, CSF had a general stimulating effect demonstrated by the faster loss of self-renewing capacity and stronger cell extension outgrowth. Adult hNSCs differentiated predominantly into astrocytes (38% in CSF, 25% in standard media) when treated with CSF and to a lower extend into oligodendrocytes and neurons. After differentiation for 7 days, we found 9% of the cells to be β-tubulin$^+$ in CSF. In standard culture media, 31% of the cells were β-tubulin III$^+$. Therefore, our data strongly suggest inhibitory effects of CSF on neurogenesis of ahNSCs, but promoting effects on astroliogenesis. Possible factors in CSF influencing differentiation behaviour of NSCs are bone morphogenetic proteins (BMPs): Monoclonal antibodies against BMP7 were for example shown to inhibit CSF induced dendritic outgrowth of neurons. BMP4 was shown to induce neuronal differentiation of NSCs by activating the ERK and inhibiting the GSK3β pathway. Both described effects could be blocked by Noggin, a BMP inhibitor [40,41]. These described effects of BMPs, do have an influence on neuronal differentiation only in fetal NSCs from rat. Until recently, it remained elusive whether these BMPs may also play a role in the observed effects of adult human CSF on astroglial differentiation, but we could show that parts of the CSF mediated effects on fetal rat NSCs could be blocked by Noggin[31]. BMPs thus seem to be at least a part of the soluble factors in the CSF influencing stem cell behaviour in fetal rat NSCs. However, in the present work, we could not find any inhibiting effects of Noggin on CSF survival effects on adult human NSCs. This raises the question whether BMPs influence NSC behaviour only during ontogenesis and therefore have no influence on NSCs derived from the adult brain or whether BMPs might differential effects in human and rat cell systems.

It is well accepted that lumbar CSF is different from ventricular CSF because of both passive diffusion processes across the blood-CSF-barrier and suggested active secretion processes during the cranio-caudal circulation [42]. Consistently, all herein described CSF effects can only be attributed to leptomeningeal CSF. Whether ventricular CSF has similar same effects on NSC behaviour remains elusive. The use of CSF out of ventricular drainages is however problematic, as ventricular drainages are used in patients with obstructed CSF circulation (for example cerebral aqueduct stenosis) or other reasons of elevated brain pressure with defect blood-brain- and blood-CSF-barrier (for example after major stroke, after intracerebral bleedings or inoperable brain tumours). Furthermore, CSF out of ventricular drainages is often contaminated by blood and altered by inflammatory processes, which is why it cannot be used for the examination of healthy CSF effects.

Conclusions

Together, our results demonstrate that adult leptomeningeal CSF has a trophic influence on adult human NSCs: survival and differentiation into astroglial cells are promoted. Thus, our data point to a pivotal role of CSF in regulating adult neurogenesis under physiological and presumably also under pathological conditions as suggested previously [28-30]. Future experiments are warranted to determine which compounds within the CSF, besides BMPs, might be responsible for the effects on NPC behaviour. It also needs to be investigated whether there are different CSF compounds influencing the behaviour of NSCs originating from fetal or adult brain. This might give us the opportunity to influence resident NSCs of the SVZ to induce their proliferation as well as to promote their migration to pathologically altered brain regions.

Methods

Collection of adult human leptomeningeal CSF

The CSF samples were taken for diagnostic purpose from adult patients in the Neurological Clinic of the Ernst Moritz Arndt University of Greifswald by a lumbar puncture. Scientific use of CSF samples was approved by the local Ethics Committee. All patients gave a written informed consent for the diagnostic procedure. Lumbar puncture was performed by standard protocols. The final diagnosis of all patients was Idiopathic Normal Pressure Hydrocephalus (NPH). CSF was only used if all standard parameters were normal (cell count, glucose-, lactate. and albumin-content, immunoglobulin-quotient). Contamination with blood was excluded. In all patients, tumors and infectious diseases were excluded. Surplus CSF from diagnostic samples of all patients was spun down to remove remaining cells, pooled and analyzed to exclude non-sterility and presence of inflammatory markers. The pooled CSF was normal in all standard parameters; contamination with blood was excluded once again. The exact parameters were as follows: Cell count <1/μl, no blood contamination, normal protein of 369 mg/l, normal glucose of 3.6 mmol/l, normal lactate of 2.0 mmol/l, normal ferritine of 7.2 μg/l, normal albumin quotient of 5.0×10^{-3}, normal immunoglobulin quotients: IgG 2.1×10^{-3}, IgA 1.1×10^{-3}, IgM $<0.2 \times 10^{-3}$. Pooled CSF samples were aliquoted and frozen at -80° until used.

Isolation and propagation of adult human neural stem cells (ahNSCs)

Adult human hippocampal tissue was obtained from routine epilepsy surgery procedures (selective amygdalohippocampectomia) following informed consent of the patients. All procedures were in accordance with the Helsinki convention and approved by the ethics committees at the EMA University of Greifswald (III UV 77/06) and at Dresden University of Technology (EK47032006). The tissue was stored in ice-cold Hank's balanced salt solution (HBSS) supplemented with 11 mM glucose and 1% penicillin/streptomycin. In all patients, tumours and infectious diseases were excluded by means of high-resolution magnetic resonance imaging and screening for inflammatory markers. Additionally, neuropathological tissue examination did not reveal evidence for tumour formation. For expansion of neurospheres, tissue samples were dissociated using trypsin, DNase and mechanical trituration similar as described previously [19]. Several media and supplements were tested like DMEM, DMEM/F12, Neurobasal (all from Gibco), P4-8F (Athena) with and without N2 or B27 supplements (Gibco) and growth factors. Best results concerning especially the amount of primary neurospheres per dissected hippocampal tissue and the early passage propagation was achieved by Knock-Out DMEM medium, supplemented with 10% KO supplement; 0.5 mM glutamine; 1% penicillin/streptomycin (all from Gibco) and 20 ng/ml both EGF and FGF-2 (from Sigma-Aldrich)(KO/DMEM). Therefore this medium was chosen as control expansion medium. Cultures were incubated at 37°C in a humidified atmosphere and lowered O_2 conditions of 5% CO_2, 92% N_2 and 3 ± 2% O_2. Fresh medium was added once a week, growth factors twice a week. For BrdU labelling, cells were incubated with 10 μm BrdU for 72 h. For immunocytochemistry studies of neurospheres, these were allowed to attach for 2-4 h before been fixed as described below.

Differentiation conditions

Cells were differentiated by plating them onto poly-L-lysine-coated chamber slides or 6-well-plates in P4-8F (standard differentiation media; from AthenaES, Baltimore, MD, USA, the albumin-content of P4-8F of 250 μg/ml matches the normal albumin content of healthy adult lumbar CSF, the glucose content of P4-8F is in a physiological concentration of 7 mmol/l) or in CSF without adding any growth factors. Some of the differentiation experiments were conducted in the presence of 150 ng/ml recombinant Noggin (R&D System, Minneapolis, MN). For studying cell survival, proliferation and neurite outgrowth cells were allowed to differentiate for up to 72 hours, for investigating cell fate decisions for up to 7 days respectively. Half of the media was changed every third day. For investigating cell morphology, survival rate and marker expression by immunocytochemistry, the cultures were fixed from 0 h up to 72 h and 14 days after starting the differentiation process.

Immunostainings

For immunocytochemistry, cell cultures were fixed in 4% paraformaldehyde in PBS or with 4% paraformaldehyde/PBS followed by ice-cold acidic ethanol and 2N HCL for BrdU staining. Immuncytochemistry was carried out using standard protocols. Cell nuclei were counter stained with 4,6-diamidino-2-phenylindole (DAPI). To determine the self renewing potential of NPCs, Ki67 expression and BrdU incorporation were used. Ki67 is detected in the nucleus of proliferating cells in all active phases of the cell cycle from the late G1 phase though the M-phase [43,44]. BrdU marks cells within the S-phase of the cell cycle [45]. Antibodies and dilutions were as follows: rabbit anti-glial fibrillary acidic protein (GFAP) polyclonal 1:1000 (Chemicon International, Temecula, CA, USA), mouse anti-microtubuli associated protein (MAP2ab) monoclonal 1:100 (Pharmingen, San Diego, CA, USA), mouse anti-galactocerebroside (GalC) monoclonal 1:500 (Chemicon), rabbit anti-β-tubulin III (Tuj1) monoclonal 1:1000 (Covance, Emeryville, CA, USA), rabbit anti-Ki67 polyclonal 1:500 (Berlin Chemie AG, Berlin, Germany), mouse anti-BrdU 1:16 (Roche Applied Science, Mannheim, Germany) and secondary antibodies conjugated to Alexa 488 and 594 1:500 (Gibco/Invitrogen, Carlsbad, CA, USA).

For determining the survival rate during expansion and differentiation, dead cells were stained with propidiumiodid (PI) 1:50 (Sigma Aldrich, St. Louis, USA), cell nuclei were counter stained with Hoechst 33342 1:1000 (Sigma Aldrich, St. Louis, USA). Images were captured using inverse fluorescence microscopes (DMIL and DMI4000, Leica; Wetzlar, Germany).

Cell counts, measurements of neurites and statistics

For quantification of the percentage of cells expressing a given marker, the number of positive cells of at least five representative areas per experiment was determined relative to the total number of DAPI/Hoechst-labelled nuclei, or field of view in cm^2 where appropriate. Neurite lengths were measured with a semi-automatic distance measurement computer program (VisRoute®). In a typical experiment, a total number of 500 to 1,000 cells were counted per marker, and 500 to 1,000 neurites per time point were measured. The mean values of ≥ 3 experiments for each condition are given together with standard deviations. Statistical comparisons were made by ANOVA with post-hoc t-test or Dunnett's t-test where appropriate. P-values < 0.05 were considered as statistically significant.

Acknowledgements

The authors may thank all patients that gave the consent to use either tissue samples or CSF, the Department of Neurosurgery for tissue preparation, the Department of Anaesthesiology, the "Epilepsy-Centre" of the EMAU for informing the patients. The authors thank the Departments of Surgery and Clinical Chemistry of the EMAU for allowing us to use parts of their equipment. Special thanks to Sigrid Peters for expert technical assistance. JB and MS were supported by the "Department Neurowissenschaften" of the Ernst-Moritz-Arndt University of Greifswald. JB was supported by a grant of the Konrad Adenauer Stiftung. AH and AS were supported by the Deutsche Forschungsgemeinschaft through the DFG-Research Centre for Regenerative Therapies Dresden (CRTD).

Author details
[1]Department of Neurology, Ernst Moritz Arndt University of Greifswald, 17475 Greifswald, Germany. [2]Department of Neurosurgery, Ernst Moritz Arndt University of Greifswald, 17475 Greifswald, Germany. [3]Department of Neurology and Centre for Regenerative Therapies Dresden (CRTD), Dresden University of Technology, 01307 Dresden, Germany. [4]Department of Neurosurgery, Dresden University of Technology, 01307 Dresden, Germany.

Authors' contributions
JB carried out the experiments and drafted the manuscript. MK and AH participated in part of the experiments. AH helped optimizing the culture conditions. AD provided the CSF samples and supervised the quality control in the CSF laboratory and contributed to the initial study design. HS and MK performed the surgical procedures and provided the tissue samples. UR selected the appropriate patients for the surgical procedures. MS planned the experiments and performed the design and coordination of the study. JB, MS and AS performed the discussion of the study. MS and AS finalized the manuscript. All authors read and approved the final manuscript.

Competing interests
The authors declare that they have no competing interests.

Received: 9 July 2009 Accepted: 8 April 2010 Published: 8 April 2010

References
1. Sievertzon M, Wirta V, Mercer A, Meletis K, Erlandsson R, Wikstrom L, Frisen J, Lundeberg J: **Transcriptome analysis in primary neural stem cells using a tag cDNA amplification method.** *BMC neuroscience* 2005, **6**(1):28.
2. Gage FH: **Mammalian neural stem cells.** *Science (New York, NY)* 2000, **287**(5457):1433-1438.
3. McKay R: **Stem cells in the central nervous system.** *Science (New York, NY)* 1997, **276**(5309):66-71.
4. Svendsen CN, Caldwell MA, Ostenfeld T: **Human neural stem cells: isolation, expansion and transplantation.** *Brain pathology (Zurich, Switzerland)* 1999, **9**(3):499-513.
5. Bain G, Kitchens D, Yao M, Huettner JE, Gottlieb DI: **Embryonic stem cells express neuronal properties in vitro.** *Developmental biology* 1995, **168**(2):342-357.
6. Kawasaki H, Mizuseki K, Nishikawa S, Kaneko S, Kuwana Y, Nakanishi S, Nishikawa SI, Sasai Y: **Induction of midbrain dopaminergic neurons from ES cells by stromal cell-derived inducing activity.** *Neuron* 2000, **28**(1):31-40.
7. Kawasaki H, Suemori H, Mizuseki K, Watanabe K, Urano F, Ichinose H, Haruta M, Takahashi M, Yoshikawa K, Nishikawa S, *et al*: **Generation of dopaminergic neurons and pigmented epithelia from primate ES cells by stromal cell-derived inducing activity.** *Proceedings of the National Academy of Sciences of the United States of America* 2002, **99**(3):1580-1585.
8. Lee SH, Lumelsky N, Studer L, Auerbach JM, McKay RD: **Efficient generation of midbrain and hindbrain neurons from mouse embryonic stem cells.** *Nature biotechnology* 2000, **18**(6):675-679.

9. Johansson CB, Momma S, Clarke DL, Risling M, Lendahl U, Frisen J: Identification of a neural stem cell in the adult mammalian central nervous system. *Cell* 1999, 96(1):25-34.
10. Magavi SS, Leavitt BR, Macklis JD: Induction of neurogenesis in the neocortex of adult mice. *Nature* 2000, 405(6789):951-955.
11. Reynolds BA, Weiss S: Generation of neurons and astrocytes from isolated cells of the adult mammalian central nervous system. *Science (New York, NY)* 1992, 255(5052):1707-1710.
12. Rietze RL, Valcanis H, Brooker GF, Thomas T, Voss AK, Bartlett PF: Purification of a pluripotent neural stem cell from the adult mouse brain. *Nature* 2001, 412(6848):736-739.
13. Shihabuddin LS, Horner PJ, Ray J, Gage FH: Adult spinal cord stem cells generate neurons after transplantation in the adult dentate gyrus. *J Neurosci* 2000, 20(23):8727-8735.
14. Hermann A, Suess C, Fauser M, Kanzler S, Witt M, Fabel K, Schwarz J, Hoglinger GU, Storch A: Rostro-caudal gradual loss of cellular diversity within the periventricular regions of the ventricular system. *Stem cells (Dayton, Ohio)* 2009, 27(4):928-941.
15. Storch A, Sabolek M, Milosevic J, Schwarz SC, Schwarz J: Midbrain-derived neural stem cells: from basic science to therapeutic approaches. *Cell and tissue research* 2004, 318(1):15-22.
16. Pagano SF, Impagnatiello F, Girelli M, Cova L, Grioni E, Onofri M, Cavallaro M, Etteri S, Vitello F, Giombini S, et al: Isolation and characterization of neural stem cells from the adult human olfactory bulb. *Stem cells (Dayton, Ohio)* 2000, 18(4):295-300.
17. Palmer TD, Schwartz PH, Taupin P, Kaspar B, Stein SA, Gage FH: Cell culture. Progenitor cells from human brain after death. *Nature* 2001, 411(6833):42-43.
18. Roy NS, Wang S, Jiang L, Kang J, Benraiss A, Harrison-Restelli C, Fraser RA, Couldwell WT, Kawaguchi A, Okano H, et al: In vitro neurogenesis by progenitor cells isolated from the adult human hippocampus. *Nature medicine* 2000, 6(3):271-277.
19. Hermann A, Maisel M, Liebau S, Gerlach M, Kleger A, Schwarz J, Kim KS, Antoniadis G, Lerche H, Storch A: Mesodermal cell types induce neurogenesis from adult human hippocampal progenitor cells. *Journal of neurochemistry* 2006, 98(2):629-640.
20. Maisel M, Herr A, Milosevic J, Hermann A, Habisch HJ, Schwarz S, Kirsch M, Antoniadis G, Brenner R, Hallmeyer-Elgner S, et al: Transcription profiling of adult and fetal human neuroprogenitors identifies divergent paths to maintain the neuroprogenitor cell state. *Stem cells (Dayton, Ohio)* 2007, 25(5):1231-1240.
21. Bachy I, Kozyraki R, Wassef M: The particles of the embryonic cerebrospinal fluid: how could they influence brain development?. *Brain research bulletin* 2008, 75(2-4):289-294.
22. Gato A, Martin P, Alonso MI, Martin C, Pulgar MA, Moro JA: Analysis of cerebro-spinal fluid protein composition in early developmental stages in chick embryos. *J Exp Zoolog A Comp Exp Biol* 2004, 301(4):280-289.
23. Gato A, Moro JA, Alonso MI, Bueno D, De La Mano A, Martin C: Embryonic cerebrospinal fluid regulates neuroepithelial survival, proliferation, and neurogenesis in chick embryos. *Anat Rec A Discov Mol Cell Evol Biol* 2005, 284(1):475-484.
24. Parada C, Gato A, Bueno D: Mammalian embryonic cerebrospinal fluid proteome has greater apolipoprotein and enzyme pattern complexity than the avian proteome. *Journal of proteome research* 2005, 4(6):2420-2428.
25. Martin C, Bueno D, Alonso MI, Moro JA, Callejo S, Parada C, Martin P, Carnicero E, Gato A: FGF2 plays a key role in embryonic cerebrospinal fluid trophic properties over chick embryo neuroepithelial stem cells. *Developmental biology* 2006, 297(2):402-416.
26. Johanson CE, Duncan JA, Klinge PM, Brinker T, Stopa EG, Silverberg GD: Multiplicity of cerebrospinal fluid functions: New challenges in health and disease. *Cerebrospinal fluid research* 2008, 5:10.
27. Mashayekhi F, Draper CE, Bannister CM, Pourghasem M, Owen-Lynch PJ, Miyan JA: Deficient cortical development in the hydrocephalic Texas (H-Tx) rat: a role for CSF. *Brain* 2002, 125(Pt 8):1859-1874.
28. Alcazar A, Regidor I, Masjuan J, Salinas M, Alvarez-Cermeno JC: Induction of apoptosis by cerebrospinal fluid from patients with primary-progressive multiple sclerosis in cultured neurons. *Neuroscience letters* 1998, 255(2):75-78.
29. Colombo JA, Napp MI: Cerebrospinal fluid from L-dopa-treated Parkinson's disease patients is dystrophic for various neural cell types ex vivo: effects of astroglia. *Experimental neurology* 1998, 154(2):452-463.
30. Redzic ZB, Preston JE, Duncan JA, Chodobski A, Szmydynger-Chodobska J: The choroid plexus-cerebrospinal fluid system: from development to aging. *Current topics in developmental biology* 2005, 71:1-52.
31. Buddensiek J, Dressel A, Kowalski M, Storch A, Sabolek M: Adult cerebrospinal fluid inhibits neurogenesis but facilitates gliogenesis from fetal rat neural stem cells. *Journal of neuroscience research* 2009, 87(14):3054-3066.
32. Sawamoto K, Wichterle H, Gonzalez-Perez O, Cholfin JA, Yamada M, Spassky N, Murcia NS, Garcia-Verdugo JM, Marin O, Rubenstein JL, et al: New neurons follow the flow of cerebrospinal fluid in the adult brain. *Science (New York, NY)* 2006, 311(5761):629-632.
33. Alvarez-Buylla A, Garcia-Verdugo JM: Neurogenesis in adult subventricular zone. *J Neurosci* 2002, 22(3):629-634.
34. Tramontin AD, Garcia-Verdugo JM, Lim DA, Alvarez-Buylla A: Postnatal development of radial glia and the ventricular zone (VZ): a continuum of the neural stem cell compartment. *Cereb Cortex* 2003, 13(6):580-587.
35. Vigh B, Manzano e Silva MJ, Frank CL, Vincze C, Czirok SJ, Szabo A, Lukats A, Szel A: The system of cerebrospinal fluid-contacting neurons. Its supposed role in the nonsynaptic signal transmission of the brain. *Histology and histopathology* 2004, 19(2):607-628.
36. Huttner HB, Janich P, Kohrmann M, Jaszai J, Siebzehnrubl F, Blumcke I, Suttorp M, Gahr M, Kuhnt D, Nimsky C, et al: The stem cell marker prominin-1/CD133 on membrane particles in human cerebrospinal fluid offers novel approaches for studying central nervous system disease. *Stem cells (Dayton, Ohio)* 2008, 26(3):698-705.
37. Nordin C, Gupta RC, Sjodin I: Cerebrospinal fluid amino acids in pathological gamblers and healthy controls. *Neuropsychobiology* 2007, 56(2-3):152-158.
38. Bai H, Suzuki Y, Noda T, Wu S, Kataoka K, Kitada M, Ohta M, Chou H, Ide C: Dissemination and proliferation of neural stem cells on the spinal cord by injection into the fourth ventricle of the rat: a method for cell transplantation. *Journal of neuroscience methods* 2003, 124(2):181-187.
39. Wu S, Suzuki Y, Kitada M, Kataoka K, Kitaura M, Chou H, Nishimura Y, Ide C: New method for transplantation of neurosphere cells into injured spinal cord through cerebrospinal fluid in rat. *Neuroscience letters* 2002, 318(2):81-84.
40. Dattatreyamurty B, Roux E, Horbinski C, Kaplan PL, Robak LA, Beck HN, Lein P, Higgins D, Chandrasekaran V: Cerebrospinal fluid contains biologically active bone morphogenetic protein-7. *Experimental neurology* 2001, 172(2):273-281.
41. Moon BS, Yoon JY, Kim MY, Lee SH, Choi T, Choi KY: Bone morphogenetic protein 4 stimulates neuronal differentiation of neuronal stem cells through the ERK pathway. *Experimental & molecular medicine* 2009, 41(2):116-125.
42. Miyan JA, Zendah M, Mashayekhi F, Owen-Lynch PJ: Cerebrospinal fluid supports viability and proliferation of cortical cells in vitro, mirroring in vivo development. *Cerebrospinal fluid research* 2006, 3:2.
43. Gerdes J, Lemke H, Baisch H, Wacker HH, Schwab U, Stein H: Cell cycle analysis of a cell proliferation-associated human nuclear antigen defined by the monoclonal antibody Ki-67. *J Immunol* 1984, 133(4):1710-1715.
44. Gerdes J, Schwab U, Lemke H, Stein H: Production of a mouse monoclonal antibody reactive with a human nuclear antigen associated with cell proliferation. *International journal of cancer* 1983, 31(1):13-20.
45. Eisch AJ, Mandyam CD: Adult neurogenesis: can analysis of cell cycle proteins move us "Beyond BrdU"? *Current pharmaceutical biotechnology* 2007, 8(3):147-165.

doi:10.1186/1471-2202-11-48
Cite this article as: Buddensiek et al.: Cerebrospinal fluid promotes survival and astroglial differentiation of adult human neural progenitor cells but inhibits proliferation and neuronal differentiation. *BMC Neuroscience* 2010 11:48.

i want morebooks!

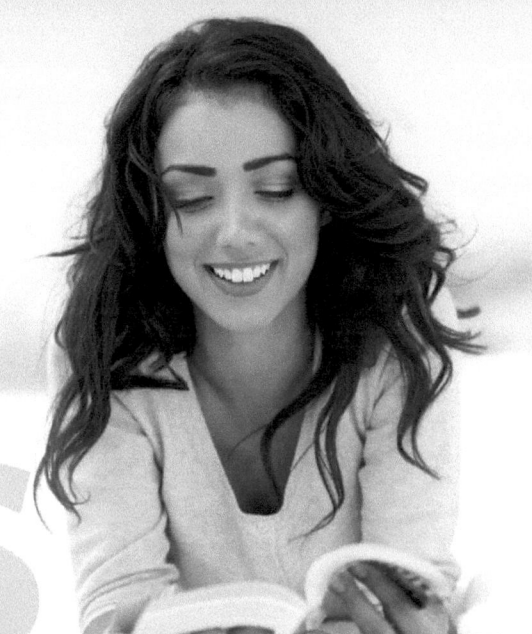

Buy your books fast and straightforward online - at one of world's fastest growing online book stores! Environmentally sound due to Print-on-Demand technologies.

Buy your books online at
www.get-morebooks.com

Kaufen Sie Ihre Bücher schnell und unkompliziert online – auf einer der am schnellsten wachsenden Buchhandelsplattformen weltweit! Dank Print-On-Demand umwelt- und ressourcenschonend produziert.

Bücher schneller online kaufen
www.morebooks.de

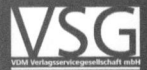

VDM Verlagsservicegesellschaft mbH
Heinrich-Böcking-Str. 6-8   Telefon: +49 681 3720 174   info@vdm-vsg.de
D - 66121 Saarbrücken   Telefax: +49 681 3720 1749   www.vdm-vsg.de

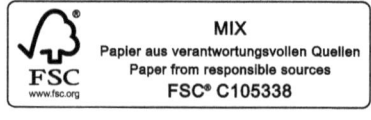

Printed by Books on Demand GmbH, Norderstedt / Germany